Reproductive Endocrinology and Infertility

Editors

AMANDA J. ADELEYE
ALBERUNI MUSA ZAMAH

OBSTETRICS AND GYNECOLOGY CLINICS OF NORTH AMERICA

www.obgyn.theclinics.com

Consulting Editor
WILLIAM F. RAYBURN

December 2023 • Volume 50 • Number 4

ELSEVIER

1600 John F. Kennedy Boulevard • Suite 1800 • Philadelphia, Pennsylvania, 19103-2899

http://www.theclinics.com

OBSTETRICS AND GYNECOLOGY CLINICS OF NORTH AMERICA Volume 50 Number 4
December 2023 ISSN 0889-8545, ISBN-13: 978-0-443-18296-9

Editor: Kerry Holland
Developmental Editor: Hannah Almira Lopez

Obstetrics and Gynecology Clinics (ISSN 0889-8545) is published quarterly by Elsevier Inc., 360 Park Avenue South, New York, NY 10010-1710. Months of issue are March, June, September, and December. Periodicals postage paid at New York, NY, and additional mailing offices. Subscription price per year is $355.00 (US individuals), $757.00 (US institutions), $100.00 (US students), $428.00 (Canadian individuals), $956.00 (Canadian institutions), $100.00 (Canadian students), $487.00 (international individuals), $956.00 (international institutions), and $225.00 (international students). To receive student/resident rate, orders must be accompanied by name of affiliated institution, date of term, and the signature of program/residency coordinator on institution letterhead. Orders will be billed at individual rate until proof of status is received. Foreign air speed delivery is included in all *Clinics* subscription prices. All prices are subject to change without notice. POSTMASTER: Send address changes to *Obstetrics and Gynecology Clinics*, Elsevier Health Sciences Division, Subscription Customer Service, 3251 Riverport Lane, Maryland Heights, MO 63043. **Customer Service: Telephone: 1-800-654-2452 (U.S. and Canada); 314-447-8871 (outside U.S. and Canada). Fax: 314-447-8029. E-mail: journalscustomerservice-usa@elsevier.com (for print support); journalsonlinesupport-usa@elsevier.com (for online support).**

Reprints. For copies of 100 or more of articles in this publication, please contact the Commercial Reprints Department, Elsevier Inc., 360 Park Avenue South, New York, New York 10010-1710. Tel.: 212-633-3874; Fax: 212-633-3820; E-mail: reprints@elsevier.com.

Obstetrics and Gynecology Clinics of North America is also published in Spanish by McGraw-Hill Interamericana Editores S.A., P.O. Box 5-237, 06500, Mexico; in Portuguese by Reichmann and Affonso Editores, Rio de Janeiro, Brazil; and in Greek by Paschalidis Medical Publications, Athens, Greece.

Obstetrics and Gynecology Clinics of North America is covered in MEDLINE/PubMed (Index Medicus), Excerpta Medica, Current Concepts/Clinical Medicine, Science Citation Index, BIOSIS, CINAHL, and ISI/BIOMED.

Contributors

CONSULTING EDITOR

WILLIAM F. RAYBURN, MD, MBA
Affiliate Professor, Department of Obstetrics and Gynecology and College of Graduate Studies, Medical University of South Carolina Charleston, South Carolina; Emeritus Distinguished Professor, Department of Obstetrics and Gynecology, University of New Mexico School of Medicine, Albuquerque, New Mexico

EDITORS

AMANDA J. ADELEYE, MD
Assistant Professor, Department of Obstetrics and Gynecology, The University of Chicago, Chicago, Illinois, USA

ALBERUNI MUSA ZAMAH, MD, PhD
Associate Professor, Department of Obstetrics and Gynecology, The University of Chicago, Chicago, Illinois, USA

AUTHORS

SAMAR ALKHRAIT, MD
Department of Obstetrics and Gynecology, University of Chicago Medicine, Chicago, Illinois, USA

CHRISTINA E. BOOTS, MD, MSCI
Associate Professor of Obstetrics and Gynecology, Division of Reproductive Endocrinology and Infertility, Northwestern University Feinberg School of Medicine, Chicago, Illinois, USA

MAXWELL EDMONDS, MD, PhD
Department of Obstetrics and Gynecology, Duke University School of Medicine, Durham, North Carolina, USA

NICOLÁS OMAR FRANCONE, MD
McGaw Medical Center of Northwestern University, Division of Reproductive Endocrinology and Infertility, Northwestern University Feinberg School of Medicine, Chicago, Illinois, USA

DAVID FRANKFURTER, MD
Yale Medical School, Department of Obstetrics, Gynecology and Reproductive Sciences, Yale Fertility Center, Orange, Connecticut, USA

EDUARDO HARITON, MD, MBA
Reproductive Science Center of the San Francisco Bay Area, San Ramon, California, USA

TARUN JAIN, MD
Division of Reproductive Endocrinology and Infertility, Department of Obstetrics and Gynecology, Northwestern University Feinberg School of Medicine, Chicago, Illinois, USA

VICTORIA S. JIANG, MD
Division of Reproductive Endocrinology and Infertility, Vincent Department of Obstetrics and Gynecology, Massachusetts General Hospital, Harvard Medical School, Boston, Massachusetts, USA

PATRICIA T. JIMENEZ, MD
Department of Obstetrics and Gynecology, Division of Reproductive Endocrinology and Infertility, Washington University, St Louis, Missouri, USA

HARVEY KLIMAN, MD, PhD
Yale School of Medicine, Kliman Laboratories, Reproductive and Placental Research Unit, Department of Obstetrics, Gynecology and Reproductive Sciences, New Haven, Connecticut, USA

ALYSSA K. KOSTURAKIS, MD, MS
Department of Obstetrics and Gynecology, University of Washington, Seattle, Washington, USA

HERNAN LESCAY, MD
Department of Surgery, Section of Urology, University of Chicago Medicine, Chicago, Illinois, USA

OBIANUJU SANDRA MADUEKE-LAVEAUX, MD, MPH
Department of Obstetrics and Gynecology, University of Chicago Medicine, Chicago, Illinois, USA

IANA MALASEVSKAIA, MD
Private Clinic of Obstetrics and Gynecology, Sana'a, Republic of Yemen

SLOANE MEBANE, MD
Department of Obstetrics and Gynecology, Duke University School of Medicine, Durham, North Carolina, USA

TICARA L. ONYEWUENYI, MD, MPH
Department of Obstetrics and Gynecology, Kaiser Permanente Northern California, Oakland, California, USA

ZORAN J. PAVLOVIC, MD
Department of Obstetrics and Gynecology/Reproductive Endocrinology and Infertility, University of South Florida, Morsani College of Medicine, Tampa, Florida, USA

BENJAMIN J. PEIPERT, MD
Division of Reproductive Endocrinology and Infertility, Hospital of the University of Pennsylvania, Philadelphia, Pennsylvania, USA

AILEEN PORTUGAL, MD
Department of Obstetrics and Gynecology, University of California, San Francisco, San Francisco, California, USA; Department of Obstetrics and Gynecology, Division of Reproductive Endocrinology and Infertility, Washington University, St Louis, Missouri, USA

MOLLY M. QUINN, MD
University of Southern California, Los Angeles General Medical Center, Los Angeles, California, USA; HRC Fertility, Pasadena, California, USA

OMER RAHEEM, MD, MSC, MCH, MRCS
Assistant Professor of Surgery-Urology, Department of Surgery, Section of Urology, University of Chicago Medicine, Chicago, Illinois, USA

NIHAR RAMA, BS
Pritzker School of Medicine, University of Chicago, Chicago, Illinois, USA

TIA RAMIREZ, MD
McGaw Medical Center of Northwestern University, Division of Reproductive Endocrinology and Infertility, Northwestern University Feinberg School of Medicine, Chicago, Illinois, USA

GREYSHA RIVERA-CRUZ, MD
IVF Florida Reproductive Associates, Herbert Wertheim College Medicine, Florida International University, Margate, Florida, USA

BONNIE B. SONG, MD
University of Southern California, Los Angeles General Medical Center, Los Angeles, California, USA

LAUREN VERRILLI, MD, MSCI
Assistant Professor, Department of Obstetrics and Gynecology, University of Utah School of Medicine, Salt Lake City, Utah, USA

LESTER WATCH, MD
Department of Obstetrics and Gynecology, Duke University School of Medicine, Durham, North Carolina, USA

Contents

Foreword: Addressing the Increased Demand for Fertility Services   xi

William F. Rayburn

Preface: The Future of Fertility Care   xiii

Amanda J. Adeleye and Alberuni Musa Zamah

Primary Ovarian Insufficiency and Ovarian Aging   653

Lauren Verrilli

> Primary ovarian insufficiency (POI) is a complex condition of aberrant ovarian aging. POI etiologies are varied, and most cases have no identifiable underlying cause. Caring for women with POI requires an approach that understands the importance of ovarian function in a variety of target organs and tissues.

Fibroids and Fertility   663

Samar Alkhrait, Iana Malasevskaia, and Obianuju Sandra Madueke-Laveaux

> Uterine fibroids significantly impact women's reproductive health, influencing fertility potential and pregnancy outcomes. Their growth, often facilitated by hormonal influences like estrogen and progesterone, can cause considerable disruptions in the uterus, leading to symptoms and complications that impact the quality of life and reproductive prospects of women. This article provides an exhaustive discussion of uterine fibroids, including pathophysiology, their impact on endometrial function, receptivity, fertility, and pregnancy outcomes, and the management of infertility in patients with uterine fibroids. It underlines the critical role of uterine fibroids in women's reproductive health, emphasizing the importance of effective diagnosis and treatment to promote fertility and improve pregnancy outcomes.

Progress on the Endometrium   677

David Frankfurter and Harvey Kliman

> The endometrium is a dynamic tissue that facilitates mammalian internal reproduction and thus, the ability to deliver live born progeny that are more easily protected from predators. This tissue is unique in its ability to undergo cyclic regeneration and destruction in the absence of pregnancy. Ovarian steroids guide endometrial proliferation and maturation promoting its receptivity and selectivity with regards to blastocyst implantation. It is decidualization, terminal stromal maturation, that prevents the trophoblast from breeching containment of the uterus and allows for endometrial sloughing should pregnancy not occur. Endometrial pathology is highly variable and therefore a wide array of diagnostic measures are required for its interrogation. There remains no single test that can distinguish between all potential issues and it is critical that appropriate and evidence-based endometrial assessment is carried out. Emerging data

on developmental markers, inflammatory mediators, and bacterial profiling offer hope that conditions including endometriosis, cancer, infertility, and implantation failure will be more easily and less invasively diagnosed. This will allow for a more timely and targeted approach to intervention. Accordingly, assessing novel measures requires an evidence-based approach prior to their mass utilization.

Contemporary Management of the Patient with Polycystic Ovary Syndrome   695

Nicolás Omar Francone, Tia Ramirez, and Christina E. Boots

Polycystic ovary syndrome (PCOS) is a complex syndrome that affects menstrual regularity, causes hyperandrogenism, increases the risk of metabolic dysfunction and infertility, and is associated with higher rates of mental health disorders. The symptoms of PCOS are unique to each individual and will evolve throughout their reproductive lifespan and beyond. Thus, care should be personalized and provided by an appropriate team of multidisciplinary physicians and clinicians, such as dieticians and psychologists.

Planned Oocyte Cryopreservation: A Review of Current Evidence on Outcomes, Safety and Risks   707

Bonnie B. Song and Molly M. Quinn

Although oocyte cryopreservation was initially used as a fertility preservation strategy for medical indications, it is now is increasingly used to circumvent age-related infertility. Outcomes following planned oocyte vitrification, also known as elective egg freezing, are limited. Current studies show higher success rates for individuals undergoing fertility preservation treatment under age 35. Additionally, while freezing 20 oocytes is optimal to achieve pregnancy, freezing at least 8-10 oocytes is recommended. While fertility is not guaranteed, current evidence demonstrates that planned oocyte vitrification is an overall safe, low risk method of fertility preservation to reduce the risk for age-related infertility.

Economics of Fertility Care   721

Benjamin J. Peipert, Sloane Mebane, Maxwell Edmonds, Lester Watch, and Tarun Jain

Family building is a human right. The high cost and lack of insurance coverage associated with fertility treatments in the United States have made treatment inaccessible for many patients. The universal uptake of "add-on" services has further contributed to high out-of-pocket costs. Expansion in access to infertility care has occurred in several states through implementation of insurance mandates, and more employers are offering fertility benefits to attract and retain employees. An understanding of the economic issues shaping fertility should inform future policies aimed at promoting evidence-based practices and improving access to care in the United States.

Breaking Down Barriers: Advancing Toward Health Equity in Fertility Care for Black and Hispanic Patients   735

Aileen Portugal, Alyssa K. Kosturakis, Ticara L. Onyewuenyi, Greysha Rivera-Cruz, and Patricia T. Jimenez

Infertility can affect all people, regardless of race, ethnicity, or socioeconomic status. Barriers to quality fertility care include access, financial limitations, education, and social stigmas. Although racial disparities in outcomes of assisted reproductive technology can be largely attributed to the influences of systemic racism (not race), we can make changes to improve equity of care. We propose strategies in the areas of advocacy, clinical setting, community, and outcomes to address the racial disparities.

The Role of Artificial Intelligence and Machine Learning in Assisted Reproductive Technologies   747

Victoria S. Jiang, Zoran J. Pavlovic, and Eduardo Hariton

Artificial intelligence (AI) and machine learning, the form most commonly used in medicine, offer powerful tools utilizing the strengths of large data sets and intelligent algorithms. These systems can help to revolutionize delivery of treatments, access to medical care, and improvement of outcomes, particularly in the realm of reproductive medicine. Whether that is more robust oocyte and embryo grading or more accurate follicular measurement, AI will be able to aid clinicians, and most importantly patients, in providing the best possible and individualized care. However, despite all of the potential strengths of AI, algorithms are not immune to bias and are vulnerable to the many socioeconomic and demographic biases that current healthcare systems suffer from. Wrong diagnoses as well is furthering of healthcare discrimination are real possibilities if both the capabilities and limitations of AI are not well understood. Armed with appropriate knowledge of how AI can most appropriately operate within medicine, and specifically reproductive medicine, will enable clinicians to both create and utilize machine learning-based innovations for the furthering of reproductive medicine and ultimately achieving the goal of building of healthy families.

Male Factor Infertility: What Every OB/GYN Should Know   763

Nihar Rama, Hernan Lescay, and Omer Raheem

Male factor infertility plays a role in approximately 30% of infertility cases. Various causes of male factor infertility exist including congenital, acquired, idiopathic, or environmental factors. Identifying the underlying etiology of male factor infertility is a key step toward providing appropriate counseling, effective treatment options, and improving outcomes for couples with infertility. Although the recent advances and developments in assisted reproductive technology have undoubtedly improved fertility outcomes, clinicians must understand the scope of reproductive urologists in the evaluation and treatment of male infertility to provide comprehensive counseling, appropriate referral, comprehensive evaluation, and correct surgical sperm retrieval techniques when needed.

Reproductive Endocrinology and Infertility
OBSTETRICS AND GYNECOLOGY CLINICS

FORTHCOMING ISSUES

March 2024
Diversity, Equity, and Inclusion in Obstetrics and Gynecology
Versha Pleasant, *Editor*

June 2024
Sexual Medicine for Obstetrician-Gynecologists
Monica M. Christmas and Andrew Fischer, *Editors*

September 2024
Obstetrics and Gynecologic Hospitalists and Laborists
Amy VanBlaricom and Brigid McCue, *Editors*

RECENT ISSUES

September 2023
Prenatal Care
Sharon Phelan, *Editor*

June 2023
Infectious Diseases in Obstetrics and Gynecology
Kevin A. Ault and Alisa B. Kachikis, *Editors*

March 2023
Drugs in Pregnancy
Catherine S. Stika, *Editor*

Foreword

Addressing the Increased Demand for Fertility Services

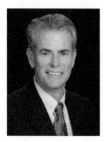

William F. Rayburn, MD, MBA
Consulting Editor

More than 10 years ago, *Obstetrics and Gynecology Clinics of North America* published an issue pertaining to medical and surgical management of common fertility issues. Since that time, demand for infertility services has grown owing to several reasons. Increased access to fertility services, a growing population, and improving success with assisted reproductive technologies (ARTs) come to mind. This increased need has led to an update on infertility, as coedited by Amanda Adeleye, MD and Alberuni Musa Zamah, MD, PhD from the University of Chicago.

This issue focuses on contemporary topics that have or will affect us all: interdisciplinary teamwork, expense of ART, financial support for expanded fertility services, artificial intelligence and machine learning in ART, improving access and outcomes for all our patients desiring fertility care, and fertility preservation strategies, such as oocyte cryopreservation.

What has remained unchanged is the prevalence of infertility using the traditional definition of infertility and when to evaluate and treat after instructing about fertility-oriented intercourse. Approximately 1 in 6 adults has experienced infertility at least once, regardless of whether they are from high-, middle-, or low-income counties. Women experience a decline in fecundity as the ovary ages, especially after age 30, so being seen in 6 months or less rather than in 1 year is standard among older reproductive-aged couples. Whether race or ethnicity impact infertility is better clarified in this issue as confounders, such as socioeconomic disadvantage and inadequate access to reproductive health services.

The couple may have multiple factors contributing to their infertility. For this reason, a complete history and physical examination and initial diagnostic evaluation should be performed. Tests to be ordered by a general obstetrician-gynecologist would include a menstrual history, semen analysis, hysterosalpingogram or sonohysterogram, and

Obstet Gynecol Clin N Am 50 (2023) xi–xii
https://doi.org/10.1016/j.ogc.2023.09.004
0889-8545/23/© 2023 Published by Elsevier Inc.

obgyn.theclinics.com

thyroid-stimulating hormone. As described in this issue, the uncertain causal relation between an abnormality on infertility testing and the actual cause of infertility makes it difficult to estimate the relative frequency of causes of infertility. Approximately 28% of infertile couples will have no explanation. This issue updates male factors, which account for about one-fourth of infertility causes.

Restricting infertility evaluation and therapy is inappropriate because of the couple's marital status, sexual orientation, or HIV status. However, an argument could be made for referral to an infertility expert. Providers with more experience in diagnosis and treatment of infertility tend to provide more cost-effective care. Such experts are also generally more able to fulfill the emotional, informational, and diagnostic needs of their patients.

Treatment involves correcting reversible causes, including lifestyle modifications and overcoming irreversible factors. Authors in this issue describe therapeutic interventions for predominantly female conditions. Descriptions of drug therapy, surgery, and procedures such as intrauterine insemination or in vitro fertilization are updated. There may be a statistically significant increase in certain pregnancy complications, such as low birth weight, preterm birth, and severe maternal morbidity, thus such complicated pregnancies may warrant coordination with a maternal–fetal medicine specialist.

I appreciate the efforts undertaken by Dr Adeleye, Dr Zamah, and their many contributors in expanding our knowledge of current topics relating to fertility care. This issue of *Obstetrics and Gynecology Clinics of North America* will be a valued addition to any obstetrician-gynecologist's library in understanding the changing landscape of basic science advances, clinical applications, and social complexities to fertility care as demand for fertility services continues. The future of infertility is multidirectional: reducing cost, avoiding complications such as ovarian hyperstimulation, and minimizing further the risk of multiple gestation.

William F. Rayburn, MD, MBA
University of New Mexico School of Medicine
Albuquerque, NM 87106, USA

Department of Obstetrics and Gynecology
Medical University of South Carolina
Charleston, SC 29425, USA

E-mail address:
wrayburnmd@gmail.com

Preface

The Future of Fertility Care

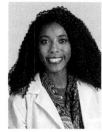
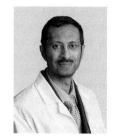

Amanda J. Adeleye, MD   Alberuni Musa Zamah, MD, PhD
Editors

Infertility is estimated to affect one in six reproductive-aged couples globally. It is critical that obstetrics and gynecology (OB/GYN) providers are aware of infertility conditions that may impact their patients and what treatments may be available to them. The field of infertility care continues to rapidly evolve; in this issue, readers will be exposed to the breadth and depth of improvements to infertility knowledge and care.

Assisted reproductive technology (ART) is a multifaceted practice and includes extensive collaboration with embryology, urology, mental health services, and more. ART, and in particular, embryology, has benefited greatly from the growth of artificial intelligence, which will be reviewed in this special issue. Urology is an important aspect of care for many of the subspecialties of OB/GYN, and infertility is no different. Therefore, it is important that providers are also up-to-date on improvements in this area, as highlighted by Raheem and colleagues.

Currently, in the United States, ART services are expensive and often unattainable without financial assistance. The financial support for fertility services is heterogenous at best and varies widely by state of residence and employment status. This has led to disparities in the access to fertility services. Jain and colleagues review the economics of fertility care, which may enlighten providers to the obstacles their patients face when they are referred for more advanced fertility services. Jimenez and colleagues review the specific issues involving the nature of racial disparities in fertility care, as well as strategies to improve access and outcomes for reproductive health care.

Uterine leiomyomas and polycystic ovarian syndrome are two conditions routinely encountered by women's health providers that often have significant consequences for fertility. Laveaux and colleagues provide an outstanding review of uterine fibroids,

Amanda Adeleye is a medical advisor and share holder for Carrot, a fertility benefits company. Amanda Adeleye has been a consultant for Flo Health.

including understanding of the pathophysiology, impacts on fertility and pregnancy, and which fibroids are best considered for surgical/medical management from a fertility perspective. Boots and colleagues summarize the major tenets of managing PCOS, including diagnosis, understanding of the individualized nature of this condition, and contemporary management strategies.

As clinicians, we are also responsible for understanding the influence of ovarian aging, not only as it relates to fertility but also for the general well-being of the women that we care for. The *Obstetrics and Gynecology Clinics of North America* had an excellent review of reproductive aging in 2018, and this special issue hopes to build upon that information with a focus on primary ovarian insufficiency. The issue of ovarian aging across the reproductive span has led many patients to consider fertility preservation strategies, such as oocyte cryopreservation, and Quinn and colleagues have provided an excellent summary of this contemporary issue.

As providers, obstetricians/gynecologists are fortunate to care for women and people across the spectrum of their reproductive lives. Understanding the landscape of fertility care in terms of the basic science advances, clinical applications, and social complexities is an important task that this special issue aims to address.

Amanda J. Adeleye, MD
Department of Obstetrics and Gynecology
The University of Chicago
5841 South Maryland Avenue, MC 2050
Chicago, IL 60637, USA

Alberuni Musa Zamah, MD, PhD
Department of Obstetrics and Gynecology
The University of Chicago
5841 South Maryland Avenue, MC 2050
Chicago, IL 60637, USA

E-mail addresses:
aadeleye@bsd.uchicago.edu (A.J. Adeleye)
azamah@bsd.uchicago.edu (A.M. Zamah)

Primary Ovarian Insufficiency and Ovarian Aging

Lauren Verrilli, MD, MSCI

KEYWORDS

- Primary ovarian insufficiency • Ovarian aging • Premature menopause

KEY POINTS

- Primary ovarian insufficiency (POI) is a distinct physiologic phenomenon from menopause.
- The human ovary is endowed with its entire ovarian reserve before birth.
- POI represents a spectrum of conditions in which the ovary undergoes a rapid depletion of a normal ovarian reserve, or has a limited ovarian reserve at birth with normal depletion rate.
- POI should be considered in women aged younger than 40 years with irregular menses, even in the absence of other menopausal signs and symptoms.
- POI has wide health implications on the female body, beyond that of reproduction. A multi-system approach to diagnosis and management is needed.

INTRODUCTION

Primary ovarian insufficiency (POI) encompasses a spectrum of disorders that ultimately lead to hypergonadotropic hypogonadism before the age of 40 years. Originally, this disorder was thought to represent premature menopause or ovarian failure; however, women with POI are distinct from menopausal women in that they may experience periods of normal ovulation and menstruation and can maintain fertility.[1] Current estimates suggest that POI affects 1:250 women by age of 35 years and 1:100 women by age of 40 years.[2] POI remains a challenging condition for patients and providers alike. It is important to understand the subtle differences between POI and menopause to be able to offer appropriate treatment and preventative care, as well as offer fertility counseling. Some of the most common complaints related to POI include infertility because it relates to menstrual irregularity, and menopausal symptoms such as hot flashes, night sweats, genitourinary symptoms of menopause, and mood changes.[3] It is important to remember the implications of estrogen in

Department of Obstetrics and Gynecology, University of Utah School of Medicine, 50 North Medical Drive, Salt Lake City, UT, USA
E-mail address: Lauren.Verrilli@hsc.utah.edu

Obstet Gynecol Clin N Am 50 (2023) 653–661
https://doi.org/10.1016/j.ogc.2023.08.004
0889-8545/23/© 2023 Elsevier Inc. All rights reserved.

tissues outside the female reproductive tract and use a whole-body approach to both diagnosis and treatment. The purpose of this review article is both to inform the reader of the physiology of 46 XX POI and possible underlying causes and to help tailor treatments based on goals of the patient.

PRIMARY OVARIAN INSUFFICIENCY PHYSIOLOGY

The human ovary, regardless of disease state or not, will undergo atresia of most follicles available throughout the female reproductive life span. The maximum number of follicles in the ovary occur before birth at approximately 20 weeks' gestation, and from this point forward, random atresia of oocytes occurs throughout the lifecycle of the human ovary, with menopause occurring when all functional oocytes are depleted from the ovary[4,5] **(Fig. 1)**. Menstrual irregularity typically precedes the final menstrual period and is thought to occur when the remaining oocytes reach a critical threshold, under which value, they will aberrantly respond to follicle stimulating hormone (FSH) and LH signaling for follicular growth and ovulation.[6] As such, POI is thought to occur either through a mechanism of accelerated depletion of the normal ovarian resting pool or through innate causes of a lower ovarian reserve at birth with normal rates of depletion.

POI is a distinct phenomenon from menopause. Although it was once called "premature ovarian failure," insufficiency is a more appropriate term because women with POI can and do sporadically ovulate, and the quality of their oocytes is more related to female age than ovarian reserve.[1,7] Important in this detail is the fact that some women with a diagnosis of POI can, and do, go on to conceive either spontaneously or with fertility treatment. Estimates of conception rates following a diagnosis of POI are poor, especially because the diagnosis may be missed or miscategorized as menopause. Current data suggest that pregnancy rates following the diagnosis of POI range from 1% to 15%, including an observational study demonstrating a spontaneous pregnancy rate of about 5%.[8–10]

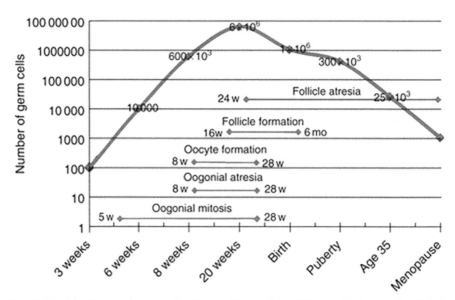

Fig. 1. The life history of germ cells. (Ozgur Oktem, Bulent Urman, Understanding follicle growth in vivo, Human Reproduction, 25(12), December 2010, 2944–2954, https://doi.org/10.1093/humrep/deq275.

The unifying physiology in POI, regardless of cause, is senescence of the function of the ovary and its response to gonadotropins, either endogenous or exogenous. In most cases, this is coupled with both ultrasound findings of limited resting follicles as well as hormonal findings of hypergonadotropic hypogonadism.[11] There are rare cases in which the ovary maintains a normal ovarian reserve but lacks the receptors to respond to FSH,[12] which is not quite within the scope of POI but manifests in similar ways.

DIAGNOSIS

The diagnosis of POI should be considered in any woman aged younger than 40 years with irregular menses. There are certain aspects of patient history that may lead the clinician toward a diagnosis of POI versus other causes of irregular menses. The diagnostic criterion for POI has classically been described as 4 months of amenorrhea in a woman aged younger than 40 years with 2 FSH levels in the menopausal range, at least 1 month apart.[3] Because the understanding of ovarian insufficiency has been distinguished from ovarian failure, the requirement of amenorrhea is no longer necessary and irregular menses is sufficient to initiate workup.[1]

Once the establishment of irregular menses has occurred, FSH levels in the menopausal range (per individual laboratory) with concurrent low estradiol (<50 pg/mL) on 2 separate occasions solidifies the diagnosis of POI.[13] If a woman has menses, the FSH and estradiol should be drawn on day 2 or 3 of menses. If she is amenorrheic or oligomenorrheic, a random FSH and estradiol level drawn at the same time are sufficient. Estradiol is a key hormone to correlate with FSH because an estradiol greater than 100 pg/mL in the setting of an elevated FSH could indicate an ovulatory event and should not be confused with POI. Thus, FSH without estradiol can be a common source of confusion in the initial diagnostic workup.

Once the initial criteria for diagnosis have been met, further testing should be initiated to elucidate any possible cause. In the setting of a fertility-based consult, a transvaginal ultrasound with antral follicle count may be helpful to guide possible ovarian stimulation options or ovulation induction.[14,15] Anti-Mullerian hormone is useful to highlight those at risk for POI but has been unable to identify those who meet diagnostic criterion, due to the low specificity of an undetectable AMH.[16] Patients with a very low AMH or a significantly elevated FSH level less than the menopausal range do have significantly diminished ovarian reserve and represent a group that is at increased risk for developing POI.

Importantly, no ovarian stimulation technique has proven to be more effective than placebo for women with POI.[15] The most efficacious option for family building among women with POI continues to be oocyte donation, embryo donation, or adoption.[8]

TESTING AND DIAGNOSIS

Once a diagnosis of POI has been made, it is important that to begin with basic examination, laboratory tests, and ultrasound to better understand potential causes (**Table 1**). A diagnosis of POI is a life-altering event, and careful attention and time should be taken to adequately explain the condition and delineate it from menopause for the patient. Most patients with POI will not yield any informative results on testing, with at least 70% of patients having an idiopathic diagnosis following testing.[17]

- *Physical Examination:* As most women with POI will have no identifiable underlying cause, the examination may be mostly normal or with slight abnormalities. Typically, women with 46 XX POI will undergo normal puberty and have Tanner

Table 1
Dos and Don'ts in the diagnosis of POI

DO	DON'T
Workup women with irregular menses < age 40 y	Wait until a woman has 4 mo of amenorrhea to initiate workup
Order FSH and estradiol together	Use a random FSH to determine diagnosis without concurrent estradiol
Counsel on fertility implications and send to reproductive endocrinologist if pregnancy is desired	Counsel on complete menopause and end of reproductive years with diagnosis
Order a baseline DEXA scan	Use a progestin withdrawal test to rule out POI
Initiate hormone therapy that aligns with a patient's reproductive goals	

stage V pubertal development. Some important clinical examination findings are listed below:

○ *Atrophic Vaginitis:* Prolonged estrogen deficiency may lead to atrophic vaginitis and vaginal itching, pain or bleeding.[18]

○ *Thyroid Goiter:* POI is associated with other endocrine disorders, such as autoimmune thyroiditis. A thorough thyroid examination should be performed to palpate for a goiter or thyroid masses.[19]

○ *Turner Syndrome Stigmata:* Turner syndrome is the most common chromosomal abnormality associated with the diagnosis of POI.[13] Typically, physical examination findings include short stature, wide chest, low hairline, and low set ears.[20]

○ *Ptosis:* Ptosis is associated with a rare genetic cause of POI blepharophimosis/ptosis/epicanthus inversus syndrome.[21]

• *Laboratory Testing:* once a diagnosis has been established based off hormonal testing, a series of bloodwork is recommended to identify any possible underlying causes of linked conditions.

○ *Karyotype:* Abnormalities of the X chromosome are the most common genetic abnormality in women with POI, accounting for 12% to 15% of all cases, with 45 X (Turner syndrome) being the most common cause.[22] The scope of this article focuses on 46 XX POI; however, it seems that there is a critical region on the long arm of the X chromosome necessary for the development and maintenance of ovarian function,[22] and therefore, other deletions, duplications, and mosaic Turner's could present as a more occult POI.

○ *Fragile X Mental Retardation Gene (FMR1) Repeat Number:* The FMR1 gene is located on the X chromosome. The 5' UTR contains an expandable region. Expansions in this 5' region can lead to a full fragile X mutation (>200 CGG repeats), and premutations (55–199 CGG repeats), which are associated with POI in female carriers.[23] The exact mechanism by which the premutation repeat number causes POI is not well understood, but the FMR1 gene is highly expressed in both fetal ovarian tissue and in granulosa cells, and mutations in this gene are linked to aberrant function of the ovarian pool.[24] FMR1 premutations are the most common heritable cause of POI and a family history of male relatives with autism or neurodevelopmental disorders may be an important piece of family history. In addition, women with FMR1 premutations are at risk of having a male child with Fragile X syndrome.[25]

○ *Thyroid Function Testing and Thyroid Peroxidase (TPO) Antibodies:* Many women with a diagnosis of POI will have already had thyroid function tests completed as part of their workup for irregular menses or amenorrhea. In addition, women with POI are at risk of thyroid dysfunction secondary to autoimmune hypothyroidism.[26] Due to this, women with POI should be screened for elevated TPO antibodies and screened annually for thyroid disease if these antibodies are present.[13]

○ *Adrenal Antibodies:* Adrenal antibodies (21 hydroxylase) are positive in approximately 3% to 4% of women with 46 XX POI.[27] If noted, patients should be referred to endocrinology for morning cortisol levels and ACTH stim test if there is concern for occult adrenal insufficiency.

○ *Ovarian Antibodies:* Currently, there is no reliable antiovarian antibody test to identify women who truly have autoimmune oophoritis. The current tests available have a high false-positive rate and are not recommended.[28] The 21-hydroxylase antibody remains the most useful antibody to detect possible autoimmune oophoritis.[29]

○ *Bone Mineral Density Testing:* Due to low circulating estrogen levels, and often prolonged time between onset of ovarian dysfunction and diagnosis, women with POI are at an increased risk of osteoporosis and fragility fractures than age-matched controls.[30] Baseline bone mineral testing (DXA scan) should be performed on women with POI and calcium and Vitamin D supplementation should be recommended in line with the North American Menopause Society supplementation for postmenopausal women.[13]

In most clinical scenarios, thorough initial testing will not reveal an obvious cause for 46 XX POI. There is an extensive catalog of gene mutations that are implicated in the diagnosis of POI; however, due to the rarity of these mutations, no genetic panel currently exists for the typical patient with a new diagnosis of POI. Familial POI may be encountered in 5% to 15% of cases and a thorough family history and understanding of age of menopause of female relatives may elucidate a longstanding history of ovarian insufficiency and referral to a genetics team is recommended.[31]

TREATMENT

Treatment of POI centers around replacing hormones (predominantly estrogen) to mimic that of a woman of reproductive age with appropriately functioning ovaries. Unless a patient has specific contraindications to hormone therapy (HT), this should be initiated at the time of diagnosis. HT in women with POI not only treats the symptoms of low estrogen (hot flashes, night sweats, headaches, vaginal atrophy, mood disorders, and so forth) but also aids in maintenance of bone, cardiovascular, and neurologic health.[32,33] HT in women with POI has been shown to reduce all-cause mortality and the use of it must be understood in this context.[34] Although some clinicians and patients alike may have concerns about HT, it is important to note that the results of the WHI study cannot be extrapolated to young women with POI who lack physiologic levels of estradiol.[32]

Bone Loss: As mentioned in the prior section on diagnosis, women with POI are at increased risk of accelerated bones loss, osteoporosis, and fragility fractures,[35] and this is more pronounced in women who develop POI before achieving peak bone mass.[36] A baseline dual-energy x-ray absorptiometry (DEXA) scan is recommended at the time of diagnosis but an interval at which a second scan should be performed is not established.[37] The mainstay treatment of maintenance of bone health is weight-bearing exercise, calcium and vitamin D supplementation, and systemic estrogen.[32]

The use of bisphosphonates is not routinely recommended in women with POI, due to the concern for long half-life and possible teratogenic effect on fetuses given the fertile potential of women with POI.[38]

Cardiovascular Disease Risk

Natural menopause poses an increased risk of cardiovascular events, change in lipid profiles and alteration of metabolic profile for all women.[39] Women with POI, however, have an independent increase in cardiovascular events and cardiovascular mortality above that of women who do not experience ovarian insufficiency.[40] Treatment with systemic estrogen therapy has been shown to restore brachial artery diameter and potentially improve vascular parameter and blood pressure, however, data on change in cardiovascular mortality is lacking.[41]

Hormone Therapy Treatment Options

Estrogen: The mainstay treatment of POI is exogenous estrogen therapy with replacement at physiologic doses. The route of HT is up to the patient and physician but a transdermal approach should be considered as a first option because it confers a lower risk of venous thromboembolism when compared with oral estrogen replacement.[42] The most typical starting dose for transdermal estradiol is a 100-mcg 17b-estradiol patch, changed weekly or twice weekly depending on brand. Oral estrace (17 b-estradiol) at a dose of 1 to 2 mg daily is also a suitable option in place of a patch.[32] Other options include an estradiol ring or gel. Routine monitoring of serum estradiol levels is not recommended because peaks and troughs make it difficult to establish a "normal" range on hormonal treatment.[32] Addition of vaginal estrace may be useful in women with persistent genitourinary symptoms despite systemic estrogen replacement.

Progestin: Choice of progestin replacement depends on many factors including fertility considerations and side effect profile. The easiest regimen is either micronized progestin (prometrium) 200 mg nightly or medroxyprogesterone acetate (provera) 10 mg for the first 12 days of each month.[13] This regimen provides adequate progesterone exposure to develop a secretory endometrium and protect against endometrial cancer.[43] For patients who desire contraception, placement of a levonorgestrel-releasing intrauterine device is an option. For women who desire fertility, only cyclic micronized prometrium should be used because it does not prevent spontaneous ovulation.[44] HT should be continued until age 50 to 51 years, at which point a taper or complete discontinuation are both reasonable options.

FERTILITY CONSIDERATIONS

Pregnancy rates following a diagnosis of POI are low and vary among studies. Most studies suggest that between 5% and 15% of women with POI will conceive after their diagnosis.[45] Many physiologic manipulations have been attempted to induce ovulation in women with POI, including prolonged use of estradiol to lower FSH followed by ovulation induction with either clomiphene citrate or gonadotropins. Despite these attempts, no regimen for ovulation induction has proven to be superior to intermittent monitoring for spontaneous ovulation.[15] Although attempts at ovarian stimulation and oocyte retrieval are reasonable, the overall yield of oocytes is expected to be low and female age should be considered when considering success rates from a low-yield oocyte retrieval. Most women who carry a pregnancy after a diagnosis of POI will do so via oocyte donation,[11] and it is recommended that this option be discussed with patients early in their diagnosis.

SUMMARY

POI is a broadly defined condition with many potential underlying causes. The diagnosis hinges on the premature loss of functional ovarian reserve and the sequelae of such loss. Many patients experience a delay in diagnosis, and it is important to approach the patient with care and compassion and acknowledge the life-altering implications of her diagnosis. As our understanding of the genetic, familial, and autoimmune pathologic conditions that can cause this condition improves, it is possible that in the future, we may have very different treatment options and prognoses based on underlying cause.

Prompt diagnostic testing, evaluation of bone mineral density and appropriate HT are necessary following the diagnosis of POI. In addition, a candid discussion regarding fertility options is important to help patients better understand and plan for their desired family goals. Management of POI is best done in a longitudinal and multidisciplinary setting and continued through the midlife menopause transition.

DISCLOSURES

Principal Investigator, Turtle Health; Physician Advisor, Alife.

REFERENCES

1. Welt CK. Primary ovarian insufficiency: a more accurate term for premature ovarian failure. Clin Endocrinol 2008;68:499–509.
2. Coulam CB, Adamson SC, Annegers JF. Incidence of premature ovarian failure. Obstet Gynecol 1986;67:604–6.
3. Rebar RW, Connolly HV. Clinical features of young women with hypergonadotropic amenorrhea. Fertil Steril 1990;53:804–10.
4. Baker TG. A Quantitative and Cytological Study of Germ Cells in Human Ovaries. Proc R Soc Lond B Biol Sci 1963;158:417–33.
5. Broekmans FJ, Soules MR, Fauser BC. Ovarian Aging: Mechanisms and Clinical Consequences. Endocr Rev 2009;30:465–93.
6. Rosen MP, Johnstone E, McCulloch CE, et al. A characterization of the relationship of ovarian reserve markers with age. Fertil Steril 2012;97:238–43.
7. Pacheco A, Cruz M, Iglesias C, et al. Very low anti-mullerian hormone concentrations are not an independent predictor of embryo quality and pregnancy rate. Reprod Biomed Online 2018;37:113–9.
8. van Kasteren YM, Schoemaker J. Premature ovarian failure: a systematic review on therapeutic interventions to restore ovarian function and achieve pregnancy. Hum Reprod Update 1999;5:483–92.
9. Fraison E, Crawford G, Casper G, et al. Pregnancy following diagnosis of premature ovarian insufficiency: a systematic review. Reprod Biomed Online 2019;39: 467–76.
10. Baker V. Life plans and family-building options for women with primary ovarian insufficiency. Semin Reprod Med 2011;29:362–72.
11. De Vos M, Devroey P, Fauser BC. Primary ovarian insufficiency. Lancet 2010;376: 911–21.
12. Aittomaki K, Lucena JL, Pakarinen P, et al. Mutation in the follicle-stimulating hormone receptor gene causes hereditary hypergonadotropic ovarian failure. Cell 1995;82:959–68.
13. Nelson LM. Clinical practice. Primary ovarian insufficiency. N Engl J Med 2009; 360:606–14.

14. Ishizuka B. Current Understanding of the Etiology, Symptomatology, and Treatment Options in Premature Ovarian Insufficiency (POI). Front Endocrinol 2021; 12:626924.

15. Hatirnaz S, Basbug A, Akarsu S, et al. Outcomes of random start versus clomiphene citrate and gonadotropin cycles in occult premature ovarian insufficiency patients, refusing oocyte donation: a retrospective cohort study. Gynecol Endocrinol 2018;34:949–54.

16. Anderson RA, Nelson SM. Anti-Mullerian Hormone in the Diagnosis and Prediction of Premature Ovarian Insufficiency. Semin Reprod Med 2020;38:263–9.

17. Rudnicka E, Kruszewska J, Klicka K, et al. Premature ovarian insufficiency - aetiopathology, epidemiology, and diagnostic evaluation. Prz Menopauzalny 2018; 17:105–8.

18. Faubion SS, Sood R, Kapoor E. Genitourinary Syndrome of Menopause: Management Strategies for the Clinician. Mayo Clin Proc 2017;92:1842–9.

19. Kirshenbaum M, Orvieto R. Premature ovarian insufficiency (POI) and autoimmunity-an update appraisal. J Assist Reprod Genet 2019;36:2207–15.

20. Ranke MB, Saenger P. Turner's syndrome. Lancet 2001;358:309–14.

21. Chen M, Jiang H, Zhang C. Selected Genetic Factors Associated with Primary Ovarian Insufficiency. Int J Mol Sci 2023;24:4423.

22. Chapman C, Cree L, Shelling AN. The genetics of premature ovarian failure: current perspectives. Int J Womens Health 2015;7:799–810.

23. Allingham-Hawkins DJ, Babul-Hirji R, Chitayat D, et al. Fragile X premutation is a significant risk factor for premature ovarian failure: the International Collaborative POF in Fragile X study–preliminary data. Am J Med Genet 1999;83:322–5.

24. Allen EG, Charen K, Hipp HS, et al. Refining the risk for fragile X-associated primary ovarian insufficiency (FXPOI) by FMR1 CGG repeat size. Genet Med 2021; 23:1648–55.

25. Wittenberger MD, Hagerman RJ, Sherman SL, et al. The FMR1 premutation and reproduction. Fertil Steril 2007;87:456–65.

26. Kim TJ, Anasti JN, Flack MR, et al. Routine endocrine screening for patients with karyotypically normal spontaneous premature ovarian failure. Obstet Gynecol 1997;89:777–9.

27. Bakalov VK, Vanderhoof VH, Bondy CA, et al. Adrenal antibodies detect asymptomatic auto-immune adrenal insufficiency in young women with spontaneous premature ovarian failure. Hum Reprod 2002;17:2096–100.

28. Novosad JA, Kalantaridou SN, Tong ZB, et al. Ovarian antibodies as detected by indirect immunofluorescence are unreliable in the diagnosis of autoimmune premature ovarian failure: a controlled evaluation. BMC Wom Health 2003;3:2.

29. Bakalov VK, Anasti JN, Calis KA, et al. Autoimmune oophoritis as a mechanism of follicular dysfunction in women with 46,XX spontaneous premature ovarian failure. Fertil Steril 2005;84:958–65.

30. Anasti JN, Kalantaridou SN, Kimzey LM, et al. Bone loss in young women with karyotypically normal spontaneous premature ovarian failure. Obstet Gynecol 1998;91:12–5.

31. van Kasteren YM, Hundscheid RD, Smits AP, et al. Familial idiopathic premature ovarian failure: an overrated and underestimated genetic disease? Hum Reprod 1999;14:2455–9.

32. Committee Opinion No. 698 Summary: Hormone Therapy in Primary Ovarian Insufficiency. Obstet Gynecol 2017;129:963–4.

33. Faubion SS, Kuhle CL, Shuster LT, et al. Long-term health consequences of premature or early menopause and considerations for management. Climacteric 2015;18:483–91.

34. Mondul AM, Rodriguez C, Jacobs EJ, et al. Age at natural menopause and cause-specific mortality. Am J Epidemiol 2005;162:1089–97.

35. Gallagher JC. Effect of early menopause on bone mineral density and fractures. Menopause 2007;14:567–71.

36. Popat VB, Calis KA, Vanderhoof VH, et al. Bone mineral density in estrogen-deficient young women. J Clin Endocrinol Metab 2009;94:2277–83.

37. Leite-Silva P, Bedone A, Pinto-Neto AM, et al. Factors associated with bone density in young women with karyotypically normal spontaneous premature ovarian failure. Arch Gynecol Obstet 2009;280:177–81.

38. Drake MT, Clarke BL, Khosla S. Bisphosphonates: mechanism of action and role in clinical practice. Mayo Clin Proc 2008;83:1032–45.

39. Gordon T, Kannel WB, Hjortland MC, et al. Menopause and coronary heart disease. The Framingham Study. Ann Intern Med 1978;89:157–61.

40. Atsma F, Bartelink ML, Grobbee DE, et al. Postmenopausal status and early menopause as independent risk factors for cardiovascular disease: a meta-analysis. Menopause 2006;13:265–79.

41. Langrish JP, Mills NL, Bath LE, et al. Cardiovascular effects of physiological and standard sex steroid replacement regimens in premature ovarian failure. Hypertension 2009;53:805–11.

42. Scarabin PY, Oger E, Plu-Bureau G, et al. Differential association of oral and transdermal oestrogen-replacement therapy with venous thromboembolism risk. Lancet 2003;362:428–32.

43. Jaakkola S, Lyytinen HK, Dyba T, et al. Endometrial cancer associated with various forms of postmenopausal hormone therapy: a case control study. Int J Cancer 2011;128:1644–51.

44. He Y, Wang W, Wu C, et al. Spontaneous pregnancy after tracking ovulation during menstruation: A case report of a woman with premature ovarian insufficiency and repeated failure of in vitro fertilization. Front Med 2022;9:994674.

45. Schover LR. Premature ovarian failure and its consequences: vasomotor symptoms, sexuality, and fertility. J Clin Oncol 2008;26:753–8.

Fibroids and Fertility

Samar Alkhrait, MD[a], Iana Malasevskaia, MD[b],
Obianuju Sandra Madueke-Laveaux, MD, MPH[c],*

KEYWORDS

- Uterine fibroids • Fertility preservation • Infertility • Pathophysiology • Myomectomy
- Assisted reproductive technologies (ART)

KEY POINTS

- Pathophysiology of Uterine Fibroids: Uterine fibroids, also known as leiomyomas, are benign tumors of the uterus. They develop from the smooth muscular tissue of the uterus, and hormonal factors (especially estrogen and progesterone) play significant roles in their growth. Despite their benign nature, fibroids can cause a variety of complications related to fertility and pregnancy.
- Impact on Endometrial Function, Receptivity, and Fertility: Fibroids can distort the uterine cavity, disrupt the endometrium, and affect its receptivity to embryo implantation, leading to reduced fertility. Intramural and submucosal fibroids, in particular, can interfere with sperm transport and embryo implantation.
- Impact on Pregnancy Outcomes: Uterine fibroids can contribute to adverse pregnancy outcomes such as miscarriage, preterm birth, and complications in labor. The presence of fibroids may also increase the likelihood of cesarean delivery.
- Myomectomy's Impact on Pregnancy Outcomes: Myomectomy, the surgical removal of fibroids, can improve fertility rates and pregnancy outcomes in some women. However, the surgery carries risks, including potential damage to the uterus, which could affect future pregnancies.
- Management of Infertility Patients with Uterine Fibroids: Management strategies include monitoring small, asymptomatic fibroids; medical therapy to reduce fibroid size and symptoms; surgical intervention for symptomatic fibroids affecting fertility; and the use of assisted reproductive technology.

INTRODUCTION AND BACKGROUND

Uterine fibroids (UFs), also known as leiomyomas, are non-cancerous growths that have been known to medical practitioners since ancient times. Hippocrates and Galen described them as "uterine stones" and "scleromas," respectively. In the 1800s, Rokitansky and Klob introduced the term "fibroid," however, Virchow recognized that they

[a] Department of OBGYN, University of Chicago Medicine, OBGYN/N101, 5841 South Maryland Avenue, Chicago, IL 60637, USA; [b] Private Clinic of Obstetrics and Gynecology, Asbahi Street, Sana'a, Republic of Yemen; [c] Department of OBGYN, University of Chicago Medicine, 5841 South Maryland Avenue, MC 2050, Chicago, IL 60637, USA
* Corresponding author.
E-mail address: slaveaux@bsd.uchicago.edu

Obstet Gynecol Clin N Am 50 (2023) 663–675
https://doi.org/10.1016/j.ogc.2023.08.006
0889-8545/23/© 2023 Elsevier Inc. All rights reserved.

obgyn.theclinics.com

stemmed from the uterus's smooth muscle tissue. The more prevalent clinical term for uterine fibroids is "myoma".[1,2]

The clinical significance of intramural fibroids on infertility is controversial, however, submucosal leiomyomas have a strong association with infertility.[3] By proactively addressing certain fibroids, individuals may experience a notable improvement in their fertility prospects. Recent years have witnessed remarkable progress in the field of fibroid treatment, offering patients an array of options compatible with preserving their fertility.

UFs can cause a variety of symptoms, including heavy menstrual bleeding, pain, and infertility. The condition can cause a significant burden on women's health, both physically and emotionally. The increasing prevalence and incidence of UFs is a global health concern. A study published in the BMC Public Health found that the prevalence of UFs increased from 126.41 million to 226.05 million between 1990 and 2019. The incidence of UFs increased from 5.77 million to 9.64 million over the same period.[4]

UFs affect up to 80% of premenopausal women. However, they often go undetected, and only about 25% of women experience any symptoms. Black women are more likely to develop UFs than women of other races. The estimated cumulative incidence of fibroids in women ≤50 year old is significantly higher for black (>80%) versus white women (~70%).[5]

In the United States, the annual cost of healthcare related to UFs is estimated to be $34.4 billion, $348 million in Germany, $120 million in France, and $86 million in England. In the United States the cost related to UFs is higher than the annual cost of breast cancer and ovarian cancer. The indirect costs of UFs, such as lost income from time off work and disability, are estimated to be an additional $1.6 to $17.2 billion annually.[4]

Historically, fibroids are classified by their location in the uterus relative to the endometrium, myometrium, and serosa (**Fig. 1**). The impact of fibroids on fertility is commonly understood and discussed based on the location of the fibroid in the uterus, as well as the size of the fibroid. The FIGO classification system (**Table 1**) is a widely used system for classifying UFs based on their location. It was developed for clinical and research purposes. However, when it comes to the practical implementation of the FIGO classification in clinical settings, experts exhibit significant divergence and lack consensus regarding agreement.[6]

PATHOPHYSIOLOGY OF UTERINE FIBROIDS

UFs develop from a single fibroid stem cell in the myometrium and are monoclonal in nature.[7] Within UFs, there are three types of cells: fully differentiated fibroid smooth muscle cells, intermediate cells, and fibroid stem cells. The presence of fibroid stem cells is crucial for the growth and expansion of these tumors.[8]

Myometrial stem cells are susceptible to genetic mutations, which can lead to the formation of fibroid stem cells, initiating tumor growth. The occurrence of fibroid stem cells is believed to be linked to genetic alterations in myometrial stem cells, such as point mutations in the mediator complex subunit 12 (MED12) gene or chromosomal rearrangements that affect the high-mobility group AT-hook 2 (HMGA2) gene. The occurrence of fibroid stem cells is believed to be linked to chromosomal rearrangements involving HMGA2 on chromosome 12's long arm, especially in larger tumors. Moreover, certain MED12 mutations found in fibroid stem cells have not been observed in the myometrial stem cell population.[9] Studies have demonstrated that the introduction of a MED12 mutation into murine uterine tissue produces tumors comparable to fibroids. These findings suggest that genetic changes may play a crucial role in the development and progression of fibroid tumors.[10]

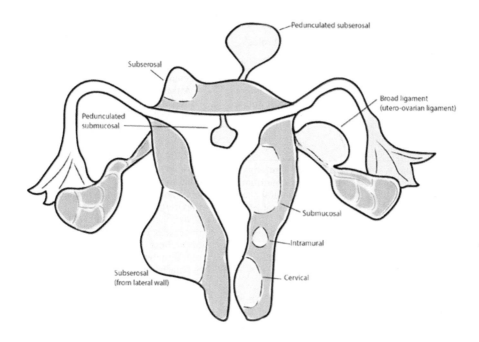

Uterine Fibroids

Fig. 1. UFs different locations.

The Wingless/Integrated/β-catenin (WNT/β-catenin) pathway promotes fibroid growth by increasing nuclear β-catenin levels. Activation of the WNT/β-catenin pathway also elevates Transforming Growth Factor β3 (TGF-β3) levels, which are higher in fibroid cells than myometrial cells due to steroid exposure. Furthermore, TGF-β3 plays a crucial role in cell proliferation and extracellular matrix deposition. It exerts paracrine effects on endometrial stromal cells (ESCs) and epithelial cells by stimulating their migration toward fibroids[9,11] **Fig. 2**.

Hormonal factors such as estrogen and progesterone play a role in promoting the proliferation of UFs, but interestingly, low levels of estrogen and progesterone receptors are expressed on fibroid stem cells suggesting that steroid hormones exert their effects on these tumor-initiating cells through paracrine mechanisms rather than direct binding.[9,12] Ethnic and environmental factors such as endocrine-disrupting chemicals (EDCs) may also contribute to tumorigenesis.[13] Recent studies have expanded our understanding of the pathogenomics of UFs including parental cells, gene networks, intergenic interactions, and driver mutations. Candidate genes for fibroid and unfavorable minor allele combinations can help assess risk factors and develop early prevention methods for UFs.[14]

THE IMPACT OF UTERINE FIBROIDS ON ENDOMETRIAL FUNCTION, RECEPTIVITY, AND FERTILITY

The pathogenesis of UFs is multifactorial and not fully understood. Abnormal expressions of extracellular matrix, growth factors, cytokines, and chemokines have been implicated in their development. Clinical manifestations are related to the number,

Table 1
FIGO classification system for uterine fibroids[5]

Location	FIGO Type	Description
Submucosal	• Type 0 • Type 1: <50% intramural • Type 2: ≥50% intramural	• 0-Pedunculated intracavitary • 1- Attached to the endometrium, but less than half of the fibroid is in the wall of the uterus • 2- Attached to the endometrium, and more than half of the fibroid is in the wall of the uterus
Other groups	• Type 3: 100% intramural, contacts endometrium • Type 4: intramural • Type 5: subserosal ≥50% intramural • Type 6: subserosal <50% intramural • Type 7: subserosal pedunculated • Type 8: other	• 3%–100% intramural; contacts endometrium • 4- Completely within the wall of the uterus • 5- Attached to the outer wall of the uterus, and more than half of the fibroid is outside the wall of the uterus • 6- Attached to the outer wall of the uterus, and less than half of the fibroid is outside the wall of the uterus • 7- Attached to the outer wall of the uterus by a stalk, and completely outside the wall of the uterus • 8- for example, cervical, parasitic
Hybrid leiomyoma group	• Two numbers listed separately separated by a hyphen with the first number indicating the endometrial relationship and the second number the serosal relationship	• Fibroids that impact both the endometrium and serosa

volume, and location of fibroids, particularly submucosal fibroids which are associated with important clinical manifestations. The "endometrial-sub endometrial myometrium unit disruption disease" has been proposed as a new entity that involves pathologic thickening or abnormality of the sub-endometrial myometrium which could be a possible site for the origin of submucosal and intramural fibroids.[15] Recent findings suggest that there are similarities between myomatosis and adenomyosis in terms of pathogenesis including inflammation,[16] endothelial nitric oxide synthesis upregulation, matrix metalloproteinase activation (MMP activation), interleukin-1 release and tumor necrosis factor-alpha (TNF-α) secretion, which could negatively impact the embryonic development and implantation. Endo myometrial junction disruption may play an important role in infertility related to fibroids as well as uterine bleeding and the growth of submucosal or intramural myomas.[15]

According to Rackow and Taylor's study (2010), homeobox protein Hox-A10 (HOXA-10) and HOXA11 mRNA expression were reduced in uteri with submucosal myomas compared to controls with normal uterine cavity and those with intramural fibroids. The authors also found a trend toward decreased endometrial HOXA10 mRNA and stromal protein expression in the intramural myoma group when compared to the control group. It is worth noting that HOXA-10 is considered one of the most recognized signaling event sequences during implantation.[17]

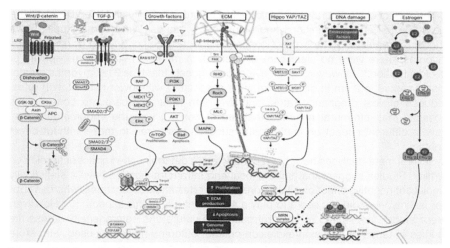

Fig. 2. Critical pathways in uterine fibroids pathogenesis.[10] The WNT/β-catenin, TGF-β,growth factor-regulated signaling, ECM,estrogen signaling, YAP/TAZ, Rho/ROCK, and DNA damage repair pathways p;ay essential roles in fibroids formation and development.In addition, the crosstalk and interaction among these pathways may initiate and trigger uterine fibroids pathogenesis. AKT, protein kinase B; APC, adenomatous polyposis coli; Bad, BCL2 associated agonist of cell death; CK1α,casein kinase 1alpha; E2, estrogen; ECM, extracellular matrix; ERE, estrogen-responsive elements; ERK, extracellular-signal-regulated kinase; ERα/β, estrogen receptor alpha/beta; FAK, focal adhesion kinase; GSK-3β, glycogen synthase kinase 3 beta; Hsp90, heat shock protein 90; LRP, lipoprotein receptor-related protein; MAPK, mitogen-activated protein kinase; MEK, mitogen-activated protein kinase kinase; mER, membrane-bound estrogen; MLC, myosin regulatory light chain 2; MRN, Mre11-Rad50-Nbs1 complex; mTOR, mechanistic target of rapamycin; P, phosophorylated site; PDK1, 3-phosphoinositide-dependent protein kinase 1; PI3K, phosphatidylinositol 3-kinase; RAF, rapidly accelerated fibrosarcoma kinase; RHO, ras-homologous; RTK, receptor tyrosine kinases; SMAD, mothers against DPP (decapentaplegic); Src, proto-oncogene tyrosine-protein kinase; TAZ, transcriptional cooactivator with PDZ-binding domain; TF, transcription factor; TGFβ, transforming growth factor beta; TGFβR, transforming growth factor beta receptor; Wnt, wingless-related integration site; YAP, yes-associated protein. (*Adapted from* Mittal, P., Shin, Y. H., Yatsenko, S. A., Castro, C. A., Surti, U., & Rajkovic, A. (2015). Med12 gain-of-function mutation causes leiomyos and genomic instability. The Journal of clinical investigation, 125(8), 3280–3284. https://doi.org/10.1172/JCI81534.)

Fibroids may impact implantation through several mechanisms, including abnormal uterine contractility, disturbances in endometrial cytokine expression, vascularization abnormalities, and chronic endometrial inflammation.[18] Submuous fibroids which are adjacent to the endometrium can produce TGF-β3 that leads to Bone morphogenetic protein 2 (BMP-2) resistance by down-regulating BMP-2 receptors in endometrial stromal cells. This mechanism is associated with reduced expression of factors such as HOXA-10 and leukocyte inhibitory factor (LIF) leading to defective decidualization and reduced implantation success.[19] Women with submucosal leiomyomas have lower levels of interleukin 2(IL-2) during the window of implantation (WOI), which could contribute to fertility issues. The presence of submucosal fibroids may also cause a blunted increase in LIF during the normal luteal phase, which has been linked to unexplained infertility and recurrent abortions. There are differences between inflammatory markers in women with submucous myomas compared to controls; however, these have not yet been correlated with pregnancy outcomes or implantation rates.[18]

The impact of intramural myomas on endometrial receptivity and infertility is still unclear due to varying definitions and diagnostic methods. While some studies have shown dysregulated gene expressions in the endometrium of women with intramural myomas, there were no significant differences in markers related to receptivity or decidualization.[20] However, recent evidence suggests that type 3 leiomyomas greater than or equal to 2 cm in diameter may be associated with lower implantation rates, reduced clinical pregnancy rates, and live birth rates compared to controls. It's possible that intramural myomas that are in contact with the endometrium may have a different impact on implantation success compared to those without direct contact.[21]

Several meta-analyses have been conducted to determine the impact of fibroids on fertility. Studies suggest that submucosal and intramural fibroids have a statistically significant negative effect on clinical pregnancy rates and delivery rates, whereas subserosal myomas did not seem to play a significant role in this aspect.[22–24] However, these studies are limited by their retrospective nature and heterogeneity across the studies in terms of inclusion/exclusion criteria, outcome measures used, etc. More research is needed to confirm these findings and better understand the relationship between fibroids and IVF outcomes. Nonetheless, it's important for clinicians to be aware of possible negative impacts on fertility when counseling patients with UFs who wish to conceive or undergo ART treatments like IVF.

While previous research has indicated that submucosal and intramural fibroids may hinder embryo implantation in assisted reproductive techniques such as IVF, it is crucial to differentiate these findings from natural fertility outcomes.

A systematic review and meta-analysis of 11 studies found that women with fibroids were more likely to be infertile than women without fibroids (OR = 3.54, 95% CI: 1.55–8.11). When specifically examining time-to-pregnancy comparisons between women with and without fibroids from the two most informative studies, the common OR was found to be 1.93 (95% CI: 0.89–4.18). However, the evidence is still limited, and more research is needed to determine the exact impact of fibroids on natural fertility.[25]

Studies suggest that the impact of fibroids on fertility potential may depend on their size and location within the uterus. While asymptomatic intramural or subserosal fibroids of size <5 cm are generally believed to have no significant impact on ART outcomes,[26] it is important to note that larger intramural fibroids (>2.85 cm) might exhibit significantly lower delivery rates when compared to matched controls without fibroids. This suggests that size could be a crucial independent variable influencing the fertility potential of these tumors.[27] Additionally, UFs location appears to be associated with pregnancy complications as posterior-located tumors were associated with more pelvic pain and higher miscarriage rates compared to anterior-located tumors in one study.[28] More research is needed to better understand how different characteristics of UFs can impact fertility outcomes in patients undergoing ART treatments like IVF or natural conception. Additionally, most studies suffer from a small sample size, potential selection bias and limited generalizability.

The systematic review and meta-analysis by Rikhraj and colleagues (2020) analyzed 15 studies with 5029 patients to determine the impact of non-cavity-distorting intramural fibroids on live birth rates in IVF cycles. Patients with these fibroids had a lower odds ratio of live birth (44%) and clinical pregnancy (32%). There was also a trend toward lower implantation rates and higher miscarriage rates in patients with these fibroids, although these did not reach statistical significance. Even a subgroup analysis of women with purely intramural fibroids showed significantly lower odds ratios for live birth rates and clinical pregnancy rates, suggesting that these tumors have a significant adverse effect on IVF outcomes in women. The study highlights the need for well-designed prospective studies to investigate whether the removal of these fibroids improves IVF outcomes in this population.[29] However, there are some limitations to this study. The study selection process may have inadvertently excluded relevant studies that did not meet the inclusion/exclusion criteria. All studies were observational, which means there could be confounding variables that were not accounted for in the analysis such as the small sample size.

In a nested retrospective case-control study, Bai and colleagues (2020) aimed to explore the impact of FIGO type 3 fibroids on IVF cycle outcomes. The study included women with intramural fibroids and matched controls, and compared implantation rate, clinical pregnancy rate, miscarriage rate, and live birth rate between groups. Women with FIGO type 3 intramural fibroids had significantly lower implantation rate (IPR), CPR, and LBR compared to non-fibroid controls. Fibroids with a maximum diameter $\geq$30 mm or multiple ($\geq$2) fibroids were found to decrease the IPR, CPR, and LBR compared with the control group while smaller ones or single fibroids had no impact on IVF outcomes. These findings suggest that FIGO type 3 fibroid $\geq$30 mm or multiple might have a negative effect on IVF cycle outcomes in women undergoing assisted reproductive techniques.[30] However, the limitations of this research are being a retrospective study, and the sample size was relatively small. The study did not take into account other factors that may have influenced IVF outcomes such as endometrial receptivity, sperm quality, or embryo quality. There could have been errors in recording information about fibroid characteristics or IVF cycle outcomes.

In summary, UFs can negatively impact endometrial function and fertility, regardless of the mode of conception, including spontaneously conceived and ART-conceived pregnancies. Submucosal fibroids have the most significant effect on implantation success. Fibroids decrease clinical pregnancy rates, delivery rates, and increase miscarriage rates regardless of location. Most studies on fibroids and fertility have been observational and retrospective, which means they have limitations such as bias and the majority were small sample sizes studies. More prospective studies and randomized controlled trials (RCTs) are needed to draw firm conclusions. The location, size, and number of fibroids may all play a role in the impact on fertility. Other factors such as age, smoking, and the use of fertility drugs should also be considered.

THE IMPACT OF UTERINE FIBROIDS & MYOMECTOMY ON PREGNANCY OUTCOMES

UFs, contingent on their location in the uterus, can significantly affect pregnancy in various ways. It's vital to understand that the uterus must provide an optimal environment for an embryo to implant and grow; therefore, UFs can lead to reduced fertility by altering the shape and environment of the cervix or uterus, which may impede sperm transport or inhibit the implantation of the embryo.[31,32] Furthermore, women with fibroids face an increased risk of miscarriage, which is thought to be connected to changes in the blood supply or the shape of the uterine cavity.[33] Submucosal fibroids, which grow into the uterine cavity, can have a more significant impact on fertility compared to those located in the wall (intramural) or outside the uterus (subserosal). Specifically, submucosal, and intramural fibroids have notably higher rates of spontaneous abortion and lower rates of live births; however, subserosal fibroids have no significant impact.[34] Multiple fibroids may further increase the miscarriage rate as they can cause a more pronounced distortion of the uterine cavity than a single fibroid, creating an inhospitable environment for the implantation and growth of an embryo.[35]

Uterine fibroids, due to their sensitivity to estrogen and progesterone, have the potential to disrupt normal fertility. Fibroid-induced distortion of the uterine cavity can hamper the process of implantation, which is essential for successful conception.

Fibroids located submucosally or those sizable enough to modify the uterine shape can particularly impede this crucial early stage of pregnancy.[34]

Furthermore, fibroids can directly obstruct the fallopian tubes, hindering the transit of the sperm to the egg or preventing the fertilized egg from reaching the uterus.[34] Even in the absence of physical obstruction, Uterine fibroids can potentially instigate an inflammatory milieu, which might detrimentally impact conception and implantation.[36] This inflammatory state can disrupt the delicate balance needed for successful fertilization and early embryonic development, adding an additional layer of complexity to the understanding of how fibroids may contribute to infertility.

Hence, the presence of fibroids can contribute to infertility through a variety of mechanisms that involve both structural and functional disruptions in the reproductive tract. It's critical to note, however, that not all fibroids impact fertility. The effect on conception largely depends on the fibroids' location, size, and number.[37] For some women with fibroids, fertility and pregnancy may proceed without any significant complications. Therefore, the decision to treat fibroids with the aim of improving fertility should always be personalized, taking into consideration the individual woman's clinical profile and reproductive goals.

Contrarily, myomectomy has been associated with enhanced fertility and improved pregnancy outcomes in some scenarios. Nevertheless, this surgical intervention is accompanied by potential drawbacks. A significant risk linked with myomectomy is the induction of intrauterine synechiae, a specific type of scar tissue formation within the uterus.

Intrauterine synechiae, also known as Asherman's syndrome, is a condition characterized by the formation of fibrous adhesions within the uterine cavity.[38] These adhesions are a by-product of uterine trauma, often induced by surgical procedures such as myomectomy. The extent of these intrauterine adhesions can range from minimal to severe, with the degree of severity having a direct impact on the affected individual's fertility.[39]

Such internal scar tissue formation has the potential to compromise the implantation of the embryo into the uterine wall, an essential step for a successful pregnancy. This could further lead to complications during labor and delivery. Conversely, scarring of the serosal layer, the external layer of the uterus, is less likely to exert significant effects on fertility.

The modality of myomectomy significantly influences the subsequent fertility outcomes. Primarily, three surgical approaches exist: hysteroscopic, laparoscopic, and abdominal myomectomy. Among these, hysteroscopic myomectomy, employed for the extraction of smaller fibroids located within or near the uterine cavity, is relatively less invasive and risky. Notably, hysteroscopy is the preferred approach for submucosal fibroids, which tend to most significantly impact fertility.[40]

Since the benefits of myomectomy may not be permanent and there is a possibility that new fibroids can develop, patients should be made aware that future pregnancies could still be affected by the recurrence of fibroids and a continued monitoring plan should be put in place. In cases where fibroids recur during pregnancy, they may not only have implications for the mother's health but can also affect the development and birth of the fetus.

Given the intricate interplay between fibroids, myomectomy, and pregnancy outcomes, it is vital for women with fibroids who are considering pregnancy to engage in detailed discussions with healthcare professionals. This includes consultations with a gynecologist, reproductive endocrinologist, and possibly a maternal-fetal medicine specialist in case of high-risk pregnancies. Being well-informed and understanding the risks involved will help in making educated decisions and developing a plan that best suits individual health needs and family planning aspirations.

MANAGEMENT OF INFERTILITY PATIENTS WITH UTERINE FIBROIDS

Management of infertility in patients with UFs necessitates a multifaceted approach that begins with an in-depth assessment. The assessment should include a detailed medical history, focusing on menstrual cycles, pain, prior surgeries, and previous attempts to conceive. A physical examination, particularly a pelvic exam, helps in evaluating the size and position of the uterus and fibroids.

Imaging studies are fundamental in diagnosing and assessing fibroids. Pelvic ultrasounds are commonly used as they are non-invasive and provide essential information about the size, number, and location of fibroids. In some cases, MRI might be used for more detailed imaging, especially if the fibroids are large or if ultrasound results are inconclusive. MRI is also beneficial in distinguishing between fibroids and adenomyosis, a condition where the inner lining of the uterus breaks through the muscle wall of the uterus, which can sometimes mimic fibroids on ultrasound. This distinction is important as the management of adenomyosis may differ from that of fibroids.[41]

The evaluation of fibroids in the context of infertility is especially important. Submucosal fibroids, which are located within the uterine cavity, or intramural fibroids that distort the uterine cavity, are particularly likely to affect fertility.[42] The number, size, and location of the fibroids must be meticulously evaluated as this information is vital for planning any intervention.

When managing infertility in patients with UFs, using Gonadotropin-releasing hormone (GnRH) agonists to shrink fibroids is often done in preparation for surgery. By using GnRH agonists, the fibroids can be significantly reduced in size,[42] which may translate to a less complicated surgical procedure.

The importance of preserving the surrounding uterine tissue cannot be overstated when the patient desires to conceive. A less invasive surgical procedure made possible by the shrinkage of fibroids through GnRH agonists can be crucial in preserving the integrity of the uterus, which in turn is essential for the implantation of the embryo and for carrying a pregnancy to term. However, it is important to note that using GnRH agonists is not a long-term solution, as once the medication is stopped, the fibroids may start growing back. Furthermore, while undergoing treatment with GnRH agonists, a woman may experience symptoms akin to the perimenopausal state, and her fecundity can often be markedly reduced or limited during this period. This alteration in the hormonal state, while not permanent, can impact the ability to conceive while under therapy.

When surgical intervention for fibroids becomes imperative, myomectomy often emerges as the fertility-sparing option. This procedure encompasses the excision of fibroids while preserving the integrity of the uterus and is crucial for women aspiring to conceive in the future. The specific approach to myomectomy—whether hysteroscopic, laparoscopic, or abdominal—depends on the size and location of the fibroids. Another treatment option is Uterine Artery Embolization (UAE). This procedure involves reducing the blood supply to the fibroids, causing them to shrink. This is achieved by injecting small particles into the uterine arteries to block the blood flow to the fibroids. However, UAE can have a negative impact on ovarian function, as the particles used to block blood flow to the fibroids can also reduce blood flow to the ovaries. As such, UAE is generally not recommended for women who want to retain their fertility unless other options are not suitable or have been unsuccessful.[43]

Assisted reproductive technologies (ART), such as in vitro fertilization (IVF), can serve as beneficial interventions in managing infertility in patients with uterine fibroids (UFs), particularly when surgical intervention is unfeasible, or fibroids do not significantly distort the uterine cavity.[44] However, it is crucial to understand that IVF primarily addresses conception issues and is generally less successful in overcoming the potential impact of fibroids on embryo implantation. Thus, even in scenarios where fibroids exist without direct distortion of the uterine cavity, a diminished likelihood of natural conception can persist, necessitating more comprehensive treatment approaches. During in vitro fertilization (IVF), oocytes are extracted from the ovaries, fertilized ex vivo, and the resultant embryos are transferred back into the uterus.[44] This technique circumvents certain challenges presented by uterine fibroids. These barriers include potential mechanical obstacles that fibroids can cause, such as obstructing the fallopian tubes or altering the uterine cavity shape, which may impede the natural journey of the sperm to the egg or the implantation of the embryo. Additionally, fibroids may impact the uterine environment, potentially affecting the endometrial receptivity necessary for successful implantation. Thus, IVF, by facilitating fertilization outside the body and subsequent transfer of the embryo directly into the uterus, can bypass some of these fibroid-induced impediments. For patients with fibroids who are undergoing IVF, individualized treatment protocols are necessary. Some patients may benefit from pretreatment with medications that help reduce fibroid size or manage symptoms. Additionally, careful monitoring during the ovarian stimulation phase of IVF is critical, as certain fibroids may respond to the hormonal medications used during this process.

Furthermore, the precise placement of embryos during the transfer procedure is critical, and in certain cases where fibroids distort the shape of the uterine cavity, a hybrid approach may be necessary. This can involve the surgical removal or reduction of fibroids followed by IVF. This is especially true for submucosal fibroids which can directly impact the lining of the uterus and affect embryo implantation.

Counseling and shared decision-making play a vital role in the management of infertility in patients with fibroids. This includes education about the condition, discussion of potential treatments and their risks and benefits, and consideration of the patient's preferences and values. The uncertainties regarding fibroids and fertility must be openly discussed.

Lastly, as fibroids can recur after treatment, long-term follow-up is crucial.[45] This involves not only monitoring for the recurrence of fibroids but also managing any emerging symptoms and continuing to evaluate fertility. Follow-up appointments should be used to reassess the patient's condition and to make any necessary adjustments to the treatment plan. As management strategies can vary based on individual circumstances, and because new treatments and protocols are constantly emerging, consulting with a gynecologist who specializes in reproductive endocrinology and fertility can provide the most current and personalized care for patients with UFs and infertility.

In light of the evidence presented, it becomes crucial for healthcare providers to recognize the significance of uterine fibroids in the realm of reproductive health. Managing fibroids with a consideration for fertility preservation should be a central aspect of care for women in their reproductive years. Patient education and involvement in decision-making are equally important, as the choices surrounding the management of fibroids can have lifelong implications. Moreover, continued collaboration among researchers, clinicians, and patients is essential for the progression of our understanding and management of uterine fibroids and their impact on fertility. Through comprehensive care and targeted research efforts, we can work toward reducing the burden of fibroids on women's fertility and improving their overall reproductive health.

CLINICS CARE POINTS

- Early Identification: Regular gynecologic check-ups can help identify the presence of fibroids early, leading to better management and reduced impact on fertility and pregnancy outcomes.
- Individualized Treatment: Management and treatment of uterine fibroids should be individualized, considering the size, number, and location of the fibroids, as well as the patient's age, symptoms, fertility desires, and general health.
- Counseling and Support: Women diagnosed with uterine fibroids should be provided with comprehensive counseling about the potential impact on their fertility and pregnancy, the benefits and risks of different treatment options, and the availability of assisted reproductive technology.
- Multidisciplinary Approach: The management of uterine fibroids, particularly in the context of infertility, requires a multidisciplinary approach involving obstetricians/gynecologists, radiologists, fertility specialists, and, in some cases, psychologists or psychiatrists for emotional support.

REFERENCES

1. Bozini N, Baracat EC. The history of myomectomy at the Medical School of University of São Paulo. Clinics 2007;62(3):209–10.
2. Singh Rahul. A Case Study of Efficacy of Homoeopathic Medicines in Case of Infertility due to Uterine Fibroid Without any Surgical Procedure. Acta Scientific Medical Sciences 2019;2:56–62.
3. Lisiecki M, Paszkowski M, Woźniak S. Fertility impairment associated with uterine fibroids - a review of literature. Przeglad menopauzalny = Menopause review 2017;16(4):137–40.
4. Lou Z, Huang Y, Li S, et al. Global, regional, and national time trends in incidence, prevalence, years lived with disability for uterine fibroids, 1990–2019: an age-period-cohort analysis for the global burden of disease 2019 study. BMC Publ Health 2023;23:916.
5. Sefah N, Ndebele S, Prince L, et al. Uterine fibroids - Causes, impact, treatment, and lens to the African perspective. Front Pharmacol 2023;13: 1045783.
6. Knipe H, El-Feky M, Rasuli B, FIGO classification system for uterine leiomyoma. Reference article, Radiopaedia.org. Accessed on 13 Jun 2023. https://doi.org/10.53347/rID-156167.
7. Bulun SE. Uterine fibroids. N Engl J Med 2013;369(14):1344–55.
8. Yin P, Ono M, Moravek MB, et al. Human uterine leiomyoma stem/progenitor cells expressing CD34 and CD49b initiate tumors in vivo. J Clin Endocrinol Metabol 2015;100(4):E601–6.
9. Ikhena DE, Bulun SE. Literature Review on the Role of Uterine Fibroids in Endometrial Function. Reprod Sci 2018;25(5):635–43.
10. Mittal P, Shin YH, Yatsenko SA, et al. Med12 gain-of-function mutation causes leiomyos and genomic instability. J Clin Invest 2015;125(8):3280–4.
11. Yang Q, Ciebiera M, Bariani MV, et al. Comprehensive Review of Uterine Fibroids: Developmental Origin, Pathogenesis, and Treatment. Endocr Rev 2022 Jul 13; 43(4):678–719. Erratum in: Endocr Rev. 2022 Mar 02;: Erratum in: Endocr Rev. 2022 Mar 02;: PMID: 34741454; PMCID: PMC9277653.

12. Andersen J, DyReyes VM, Barbieri RL, et al. Leiomyoma primary cultures have elevated transcriptional response to estrogen compared with autologous myometrial cultures. J Soc Gynecol Invest 1995;2(3):542–51.

13. Mas A, Stone L, O'Connor PM, et al. Developmental Exposure to Endocrine Disruptors Expands Murine Myometrial Stem Cell Compartment as a Prerequisite to Leiomyoma Tumorigenesis. Stem cells (Dayton, Ohio) 2017;35(3):666–78.

14. Baranov VS, Osinovskaya NS, Yarmolinskaya MI. Pathogenomics of Uterine Fibroids Development. Int J Mol Sci 2019;20(24):6151.

15. Ciavattini Andrea, Di Giuseppe Jacopo, Stortoni Piergiorgio, et al. Pasquapina Ciarmela, "Uterine Fibroids: Pathogenesis and Interactions with Endometrium and Endomyometrial Junction". Obstetrics and Gynecology International 2013; 2013:11.

16. Matsuzaki S, Canis M, Darcha C, et al. HOXA-10 expression in the mid-secretory endometrium of infertile patients with either endometriosis, uterine fibromas or unexplained infertility. Hum Reprod 2009;24(12):3180–7.

17. Rackow BW, Taylor HS. Submucosal uterine leiomyomas have a global effect on molecular determinants of endometrial receptivity. Fertil Steril 2010;93(6): 2027–34.

18. Munro MG. Uterine polyps, adenomyosis, leiomyomas, and endometrial receptivity. Fertil Steril 2019;111(4):629–40.

19. Rackow BW, Jorgensen E, Taylor HS. Endometrial polyps affect uterine receptivity. Fertil Steril 2011;95(8):2690–2.

20. Aghajanova L, Houshdaran S, Irwin JC, et al. Effects of noncavity-distorting fibroids on endometrial gene expression and function. Biol Reprod 2017;97(4): 564–76.

21. Yan L, Yu Q, Zhang YN, et al. Effect of type 3 intramural fibroids on in vitro fertilization-intracytoplasmic sperm injection outcomes: a retrospective cohort study. Fertil Steril 2018;109(5):817–22.e2.

22. Somigliana E, Vercellini P, Daguati R, et al. Fibroids and female reproduction: a critical analysis of the evidence. Hum Reprod Update 2007;13(5):465–76.

23. Pritts EA, Parker WH, Olive DL. Fibroids and infertility: an updated systematic review of the evidence. Fertil Steril 2009;91(4):1215–23.

24. Sunkara SK, Khairy M, El-Toukhy T, et al. The effect of intramural fibroids without uterine cavity involvement on the outcome of IVF treatment: a systematic review and meta-analysis. Human reproduction (Oxford, England) 2010;25(2):418–29.

25. Somigliana E, Reschini M, Bonanni V, et al. Fibroids and natural fertility: a systematic review and meta-analysis. Reprod Biomed Online 2021;43(1):100–10.

26. Somigliana E, De Benedictis S, Vercellini P, et al. Fibroids not encroaching the endometrial cavity and IVF success rate: a prospective study. Human reproduction (Oxford, England) 2011;26(4):834–9.

27. Oliveira FG, Abdelmassih VG, Diamond MP, et al. Impact of subserosal and intramural uterine fibroids that do not distort the endometrial cavity on the outcome of in vitro fertilization-intracytoplasmic sperm injection. Fertil Steril 2004;81(3): 582–7.

28. Deveer M, Deveer R, Engin-Ustun Y, et al. Comparison of pregnancy outcomes in different localizations of uterine fibroids. Clin Exp Obstet Gynecol 2012;39(4): 516–8.

29. Rikhraj K, Tan J, Taskin O, et al. The impact of noncavity-distorting intramural fibroids on live birth rate in in vitro fertilization cycles: a systematic review and meta-analysis. J Wom Health 2002;29(2):210–9.

30. Bai X, Lin Y, Chen Y, et al. The impact of FIGO type 3 fibroids on in-vitro fertilization outcomes: A nested retrospective case-control study. Eur J Obstet Gynecol Reprod Biol 2020;247:176–80.
31. Freytag D, Günther V, Maass N, et al. Uterine Fibroids and Infertility. Diagnostics 2021;11(8):1455.
32. Ali M, Al-Hendy A. Selective progesterone receptor modulators for fertility preservation in women with symptomatic uterine fibroids. Biol Reprod 2017;97(3): 337–52.
33. Lee HJ, Norwitz ER, Shaw J. Contemporary management of fibroids in pregnancy. Rev Obstet Gynecol 2010;3(1):20–7.
34. Guo XC, Segars JH. The impact and management of fibroids for fertility: an evidence-based approach. Obstet Gynecol Clin North Am 2012;39(4):521–33.
35. Olive DL, Pritts EA. Fibroids and reproduction. Semin Reprod Med 2010;28(3): 218–27.
36. Donnez J, Dolmans MM. Uterine fibroid management: from the present to the future. Hum Reprod Update 2016;22(6):665–86.
37. Stewart EA, Laughlin-Tommaso SK. (2022, November 28). Patient education: Uterine fibroids BeyondtheBasics).UpToDate. https://www.uptodate.com/contents/uterine-fibroids-beyond-the-basics/print.
38. Smikle C, Yarrarapu SNS, Khetarpal S. Asherman Syndrome. In: StatPearls Internet. Treasure Island (FL): StatPearls Publishing; 2023. Available at: https://www.ncbi.nlm.nih.gov/books/NBK448088/.
39. AAGL Elevating Gynecologic Surgery. AAGL practice report: practice guidelines on intrauterine adhesions developed in collaboration with the European Society of Gynaecological Endoscopy (ESGE). Gynecol Surg 2017;14(1):6.
40. Lasmar RB, Lasmar BP, Moawad NS. Hysteroscopic myomectomy. Medicina (Kaunas) 2022;58(11):1627.
41. Levens ED, Wesley R, Premkumar A, et al. Magnetic resonance imaging and transvaginal ultrasound for determining fibroid burden: implications for research and clinical care. Am J Obstet Gynecol 2009 May;200(5):537.e1–7.
42. Hodgson R, Bhave Chittawar P, Farquhar C. GnRH agonists for uterine fibroids. Cochrane Database Syst Rev 2017;2017(10):CD012846.
43. Kaump GR, Spies JB. The impact of uterine artery embolization on ovarian function. J Vasc Interv Radiol 2013;24(4):459–67.
44. Jain M, Singh M. Assisted reproductive technology (ART) techniques. In: StatPearls [Internet]. Treasure Island (FL): StatPearls Publishing; 2023. Available at: https://www.ncbi.nlm.nih.gov/books/NBK576409/.
45. Kramer KJ, Ottum S, Gonullu D, et al. Reoperation rates for recurrence of fibroids after abdominal myomectomy in women with large uterus. PLoS One 2021; 16(12):e0261085.

Progress on the Endometrium

David Frankfurter, MD[a],*, Harvey Kliman, MD, PhD[b]

KEYWORDS

- Endometrium • Decidualization • Window of implementation
- Endometrial receptivity • Endometrial testing • Microbiome

KEY POINTS

- Endometrial maturation allows it to become receptive to an early embryo for a limited time, "the window of implantation."
- It is the decidualized endometrium that regulates trophoblastic invasion, prevents uterine rupture, and sets the stage for placentation.
- Endometrial pathology can lead to abnormal uterine bleeding, cancer, recurrent pregnancy loss, or recurrent implantation failure and testing of the endometrium should be guided based on presentation.
- Endometrial sampling and histological assessment is helpful in assessing for hyperplasia, carcinoma, retained products of conception, and placental site tumors.
- Endometrial histology assessment for a luteal phase defect is not warranted and the widespread implementation novel endometrial diagnostic measures and/or treatments must be evidence based.

INTRODUCTION
Evolution

One of the basic tenets of biology is that living beings exist primarily to reproduce and thereby perpetuate their species. Strategies to allow for such perpetuation are variable, with viviparity among the most complex. The ability to produce live born progeny is not unique to mammals. Distinct to mammalian reproduction, however, is the placenta which provides the advantage of allowing for the delivery of live born that can be more easily protected and nourished than either eggs, larvae, or embryos alone.[1]

[a] Yale Meidcal School, Department of Obstetrics, Gynecology and Reproductive Sciences, Yale Fertility Center, 200 West Campus Drive, 2nd Floor, Orange, CT 06477, USA; [b] Yale University School of Medicine, Kliman Laboratories, Reproductive and Placental Research Unit, Department of Obstetrics, Gynecology and Reproductive Sciences, 310 Cedar Street, FMB 225, New Haven, CT 06510, USA
* Corresponding author. Yale Meidcal School, Dept of Obstetrics, Gynecology and Reproductive Sciences, Yale Fertility Center, 200 West Campus Drive, 2nd Floor, Orange, CT 06477.
E-mail address: david.frankfurter@yale.edu
Twitter: @placentatalk (H.K.)

Obstet Gynecol Clin N Am 50 (2023) 677–694
https://doi.org/10.1016/j.ogc.2023.09.002
0889-8545/23/© 2023 Elsevier Inc. All rights reserved.
obgyn.theclinics.com

The placenta provides close apposition of maternal and fetal circulations to afford the exchange of nutrients, waste, and gases.[1] Placentation requires the development and coordination of a receptive epithelium that is guided by the ovary as it repeatedly progresses from follicular to luteal phases. It is believed that the ability of the ovary to generate progesterone in response to luteinizing hormone (LH) occurred in a reptilian line that gave rise to mammals. The evolution of LH directed progesterone production by the corpus luteum provided the basis for placentation.[1]

Placentation requires the retention of a gestation in a host reproductive tract long enough to allow communication between fetal and maternal compartments. Evolutionary progression to the monotreme afforded 8 days of embryonic retention which was time enough for eggshell hardening. Obviously, placentation requires a longer gestation period as well as pituitary driven, ovarian sex steroid support.[1]

This entire process is dependent upon an endometrial interface capable of accepting and supporting the nascent conceptus. The endometrium allows for homeostasis, prevents immune recognition, and serves to temper trophoblastic invasion, thereby protecting the uterus from rupture.[2] The endometrium demonstrates a temporary receptive state termed "the window of implantation" (WOI), during which recognition, binding, and incorporation of an early embryo is possible. Implantation will not occur outside of this "window."[3,4] Should implantation not occur, endometrial denudation is required to recapitulate a receptive window—which is the basis for menstruation.[2] While the transition from a unique follicle to corpus luteum is needed to allow for endometrial development and maturation, only the endometrium repeatedly alters its biology, structure, and function to allow for viviparity.[5]

The endometrium is responsible for selecting an implantable embryo and allowing for placentation. Abnormalities in endometrial structure/function can manifest as abnormal uterine bleeding (AUB), dysmenorrhea, endometrial hyperplasia/carcinoma, implantation failure (IF), recurrent pregnancy loss (RPL), or obstetric complications.[5] The endometrium is more than a sticky permissive epithelium.[6,7] It is a complex and regulated structure that allows for the selection of a developmentally competent blastocyst which prevents repeated fetal wastage.[7] This complexity is what makes assessment, diagnosis, and treatment of an inappropriately functioning endometrium such a challenge. Endometrial dysfunction has been implicated in RPL and recurrent implantation failure (RIF). While the prevalence of RPL among couples trying to conceive is between 1% to 3%, the prevalence of RIF remains less clear with estimates ranging from less than 5% to 15%[6,8–10]. It is the goal of this review to shed light on this issue.

Endometrial Development

The endometrium derives from the mucosa of the Mullerian ducts and is comprised of 2 layers that are responsive to the fluctuations in sex steroids noted during the ovarian cycle. Following menses, the basalis layer provides the stratum for the regeneration of the functionalis layer. The functionalis mitigates implantation or sloughing depending on presence or absence of pregnancy. This process is reflected in cyclic growth and maturation. Follicular phase-derived estrogen induces proliferation which sets the stage for postovulatory, progesterone-dependent maturation. Maturation provides an opportunity for embryonic attachment, invasion, and containment. Sloughing ensues if these conditions are not met.[2,11]

As noted earlier, the purpose of this cyclic process is to open an implantation window to allow for embryonic nidation and invasion. This window is a transient entity and must close to prevent superfetation. Once closed, the window cannot reopen, and therefore, if no implantation ensues, the lining needs to be discarded in order for it to be rebuilt to reopen the window—and so on and so forth.[2,5]

Window of Implantation

Endometrial maturation involves the process by which the endometrium undergoes changes that allow for blastocyst adherence and invasion. The timeframe during which the endometrium is receptive to the attachment and invasion of a blastocyst is the WOI. This window was initially recognized when the timing for embryo transfer during in vitro fertilization (IVF) cycles was established. Transfers outside of this window did not result in pregnancies.[3,12] This was subsequently refined, and by normalizing cycle day 14 to reflect the day of ovulation, the WOI was defined as cycle days 19 to 23 of a 28-day cycle.[3,5] When considering endometrial preparation in an artificial cycle, as with a frozen-thaw embryo transfer (FT-ET) cycle, the timing of the WOI may appear confusing (**Table 1**). It can be described as the first full day of progesterone (cycle day 14) plus 5 days (P+5; cycle day 19) through the first full day of progesterone plus 9 days (P+9; cycle day 23).[5] This temporal specificity is mainly attributable to the glandular epithelium to which the blastocyst initially binds[5,13]. Because human embryos do not undergo diapause (suspension of embryonic development allowing for resumption when environmental conditions are favorable), receptivity is believed to be primarily established by the endometrium.

The process of implantation involves crosstalk between the blastocyst and epithelium. It appears that immune factors play a role in preparing the endometrium for implantation, and interestingly, paternal factors may also play a role. Maternal exposure to seminal fluid around the time of implantation has been implicated in promoting implantation.[14,15]

Implantation

Implantation involves a cascade of interactions between the blastocyst and the glandular epithelium.[5] It begins with the apposition of the blastocyst to the endometrial surface via interactions with long mucin molecules. The early embryo then tightly binds the glandular epithelium through trophoblast derived fetal fibronectin and endometrial expressed α_v/β_3 integrin. Finally, it invades into the endometrial stroma.[16] Accordingly, implantation requires that both embryo and endometrium co-develop to allow for implantation.

Decidualization

Human decidualization occurs whether or not an embryo is present, and it is choreographed by the cyclic changes that occur in ovarian steroids during the menstrual cycle.[8] While progesterone is the primary force behind decidualization, paracrine and autocrine factors are also involved. These include interleukins, leukemia inhibitory factor (LIF), cycloxygenase 2, and transforming growth factor-ß super family proteins. Taken together, they promote extracellular signaling and angiogenic regulation.[8] During decidualization, endometrial stromal cells elicit a biphasic phenotype with an initial pro-inflammatory phase followed by an anti-inflammatory response.[9,10]

In the absence of a pregnancy, the final phase of decidualization is menses, the programmed physiologic process by which the endometrium autolyzes and sloughs off when progesterone drops.[11] This is then followed by regeneration to allow for another attempt at implantation.[2,8]

Endometrial Receptivity and Selectivity

Endometrial receptivity speaks to the ability of the endometrium to allow for embryonic incursion into the endometrium. Selectivity refers to the ability of the differentiated endometrium to reject developmentally incompetent embryos. These abilities manifest as a result of hormonal signaling and cellular interactions.[17]

Table 1
Endometrium embryo progesterone testing timing

Cycle day by dating	LH Surge	LH Dating	Ovulation	Embryo Development in days and hours	Day of P exposure	P dating	EFT Biopsy	ERA Biopsy	ReceptivaDx Biopsy	Embryo Transfer
Days 1-12										
Day 13	LH surge	LH+0								
Day 14		LH+1	Ovulation	Day 0; fertilization	Day 1 (first full day)	P+0				
Day 15		LH+2		Day 1 (24 hours old); fertilization check	Day 2	P+1	d15 biopsy			
Day 16		LH+3		Day 2 (48 hours)	Day 3	P+2				
Day 17		LH+4		Day 3 (72 hours)	Day 4	P+3				day 3 embryo transfer
Day 18		LH+5		Day 4 (96 hours)	Day 5	P+4				
Day 19		LH+6		Day 5 (120 hours)	Day 6	P+5	P+5		LH+6–LH+10 or P+5–P+10	day 5 blastocyst transfer
Day 20		LH+7		Day 6 (144 hours)	Day 7	P+6		LH+7		
Day 21		LH+8		Day 7	Day 8	P+7				
Day 22		LH+9		Day 8	Day 9	P+8				
Day 23		LH+10		Day 9	Day 10	P+9				
Day 24		LH+11		Day 10	Day 11	P+10	d24 biopsy			
Day 25		LH+12		Day 11	Day 12	P+11				
Day 26		LH+13		Day 12	Day 13	P+12				
Day 27		LH+14		Day 13	Day 14	P+13				
Day 28: menses		LH+15		Day 14	Day 15	P+14				

The cycle day by dating column represents an idealized 28-d menstrual cycle. The key milestones for endometrial dating are shown in red (LH surge, day of ovulation, and first full day of progesterone). The light orange shaded columns represent the 3 major endometrial assessment tests, with the blue shaded cells being the suggested endometrial sampling days based on literature supplied by the testers. The light green shaded column matches the day 3 and 5 embryo transfers with the cycle day by dating column. EFT, endometrial function test; ERA, endometrial receptivity analysis; LH, luteinizing hormone; P, progesterone.

Luteal regression occurs in the absence of implantation. The evolutionary emergence of human chorionic gonadotropin (hCG) resulted from gene duplication (beta-hCG is identical to beta-LH except that beta-hCG has a heavily glycosylated 24 amino acid tail giving it a much longer $T_{1/2}$) and afforded the endometrium the ability to select against embryos that were deficient in hCG production.[18,19] Furthermore, in vitro modeling and in vivo data provide evidence that the human endometrium is equipped to negatively respond to poor quality embryos and favorably respond to embryos with high implantation potential.[20,21]

Decidualized stromal cells are active participants in steering stromal trophoblastic invasion and expansion. Migration of decidualized stromal cells is chemotactically guided toward competent embryos expressing platelet-derived growth factor-AA.[22] It appears that the endometrium possesses the ability to impede abnormal embryos that breach the luminal epithelium from further invasion. Further evidence of this selective ability is the finding that low quality embryos induce an endometrial epithelial stress response.[21] It stands to reason that either the loss in endometrial selectivity or enhanced endometrial receptivity may manifest in RPL while enhanced selectivity or reduced receptivity may result in infertility.[19] The normal endometrium balances receptivity and selectivity to allow for the normal establishment and progression of a pregnancy.

Implantation requires the presence of a competent embryo and a receptive endometrium.[23] A better understanding of embryo competency began with morphologic scoring, progressed through extended embryo culture, and is now assessed with preimplantation genetic testing for aneuploidy (PGT-A).[24] Previously, IVF routinely progressed through controlled ovarian hyperstimulation (COH), fertilization by insemination or intracytoplasmic sperm injection, a short course of embryo culture, and then transfer of multiple embryos in a single cycle. Rarely, IVF employed a freeze all approach whereby embryo transfer was deferred. As such, the endometrium, which developed at the mercy of COH derived supraphysiologic and accelerated hormone exposure, was largely ignored.[5] The constraints imposed by COH on the endometrium made endometrial testing implausible and endometrial sampling during a transfer cycle, in general, not encouraged.[25] Furthermore, the hormonal milieu seen with COH cannot be altered to effectively optimize endometrial maturation.

Advances in embryo culture and freezing have shifted the pendulum. That which was outside of our control is no longer so. Extended embryo culture to the blastocyst stage has become routine owing to the higher implantation, clinical pregnancy, and live birth rates (LBRs) seen with blastocyst versus cleavage stage embryos transfers.[26] Blastocyst embryo culture enables a higher likelihood of selecting a competent embryo. It reduces the need to transfer multiple embryos and provides the means for preserving high quality embryos via vitrification. The development of PGT-A augmented these features.[24] By 2015, the number of embryo FT cycles nearly matched the number of oocyte retrieval cycles in the United States.[27] IF, in the context of high utilization of PGT-A, has begun to shift the focus from the embryo to the endometrium.

Clinical Assessment of the Endometrium

Clinical presentation dictates the mode(s) of endometrial assessment. The use of the PALM-COEIN system for nomenclature of etiologies guides the tools used to diagnose AUB.[28] While the assessment for RPL includes ruling out structural uterine abnormalities including polyps and fibroids, RIF remains elusive with no clear consensus on its definition.[29] The lack of a unifying definition, therefore, leads to confusion when interpreting RIF studies. It is not unusual for those undergoing assisted reproductive technology to have negative results after multiple attempts—even with PGT-A. Pirtea and colleagues reported LBRs after the first, second, and third PGT-A derived FT single embryo transfer (SET) of 64.8%, 54.4%, and 54.1%, respectively. The cumulative LBR after 3 consecutive FT SETs was 92.6%.[10,30] This begs the question as to whether RIF reflects bad luck, and, if not, it likely has a very low incidence.[30] Because of the frustration commonly experienced with RIF and RPL, the variety and number of tests being marketed continues to grow.

Endometrial histology

Endometrial tissue is readily available for sampling and can be acquired in the office with routine sampling or in the operating room via targeted hysteroscopic biopsy or dilation and evacuation. Noyes and colleagues cemented the description of the human endometrium by providing quantifiable hallmarks of steroid-dependent, day-to-day variation in endometrial glandular and stromal histology.[31] These were the basis for defining the luteal phase deficiency (LPD). However, dating endometrial biopsies are imprecise, and LPD appears common among women with proven fertility rendering both as limitations in addressing IF and RPL.[32,33]

This is not to say that the endometrial biopsy does not provide useful information. Endometrial histology can identify pathologies, including endometrial hyperplasia, endometrial polyps, retained products of conception (rPOC), acute endometritis, endometrial tuberculosis, endometrial carcinoma, and placental site trophoblastic tumor. It may also provide evidence of for endometriosis. These findings are illustrated in Fig 4 in Kliman and Frankfurter.[5]

Excessive or unopposed estrogen, as seen in polycystic ovarian syndrome, can result in endometrial growth disorders (hyperplasia or carcinoma), and endometrial polyps may also result from hyper-estrogenemia.[34] Arresting hyperplasia involves treatment with a progestin while polypectomy can be considered for endometrial polyps.

Inflammatory lesions can also be identified histologically. The presence of neutrophils in the endometrial glandular lumen is diagnostic for a bacterial infection.[35] The presence of glandular lumen macrophages, a possible marker of the pelvic inflammation, may be suggestive of endometriosis. A more enigmatic and less common finding is an inflammatory reaction characterized by a combined lymphocytic and macrophage infiltration around and through the glands. This is not "chronic endometritis" (CE), which is considered when plasma cells are present. Instead, combined lymphocytic and macrophage infiltration is an actively destructive process that is suggestive of an autoimmune process.[5]

Finally, evidence of rPOC can often be identified via endometrial histology. The presence of persistent trophoblasts within the endometrium can interfere with normal endometrial development and lead to IF. Foci of retained trophoblasts can rarely progress to potentially lethal placental site trophoblastic tumors.[5] It should be stressed that none of these aforementioned pathologic conditions can be diagnosed without preservation of endometrial architecture. Avoiding histologic examination prevents the diagnoses of these conditions, precludes appropriate treatment, and may therefore be life threatening. However, routine histology alone cannot define the functionality of the endometrium. Functional assessment requires the identification and validation of markers of functionality.

Sonography

Ultrasound is relatively easy, safe, and noninvasive. It provides a reliable and readily available tool for endometrial assessment. Endometrial thickness (EMT) is easily measured with sonography and is felt to reflect the response of the endometrium to cycling steroids. A history of intrauterine adhesions, dilatation and curettage, uterine surgery, Mullerian anomaly, pelvic infection, radiation exposure, and in utero diethylstilbestrol exposure has been associated with a thin endometrium.[17] Estrogen-induced proliferation as reflected by late follicular EMT has been used to predict pregnancy likelihood.[17,36]

A meta-analysis representing 88,056 IVF cycles concluded that subjects with lower EMT when compared to those with higher EMTs had lower implantation, pregnancy, and LBRs. No differences between groups were observed with regards to miscarriage and ectopic pregnancy rates.[37] An analysis of all Canadian fresh and FT-ET cycles between 2013 to 15 by Liu and colleagues showed that with each millimeter decline in EMT below 8 mm clinical pregnancy and LBRs decreased while miscarriage increased in fresh IVF-ET cycles. They reported LBRs of 33.7%, 25.5%, 24.6%, and 18.1% for EMTs of more than or equal to 8, 7 to 7.9, 6 to 6.9, and 5 to 5.9 mm, respectively.[38] An analysis of over 5300 frozen-thaw cycles revealed that LBRs plateaued after EMT reached 7 to 10 mm, and that this improvement was independent of patient age or embryo transfer stage.[39]

For intrauterine insemination cycles, patients with thinner EMT had lower clinical pregnancy rates compared to those with thicker EMT. However, when 6 mm was used as the cutoff between thin and thick EMT, no difference in clinical outcome was noted.[36] Furthermore, in frozen embryo transfer cycles, those with EMTs less than 8 mm versus those with EMTs greater than 10 mm had lower birthweights (mean difference of 89–108g).[40]

While the morphologic endometrial pattern can be resolved with ultrasound, it remains to be seen whether a tri-laminar sonographic endometrial pattern is a positive predictor of pregnancy outcomes.[36] Saline infused sonography is commonly used to identify intrauterine filling defects such as polyps and fibroids.[41] The potential impact of these on live birth is felt to be a function of their size and location.[42,43] Finally, while sonography is capable of discerning gross abnormalities which may hinder pregnancy, it cannot predict pregnancy.

Natural Killer Cells

Cellular markers including natural killer cells (NK) have been implicated as potential markers of endometrial receptivity. The immune cell population changes during the luteal phase, and NK cell dysfunction has been linked to a reduction in reproductive competence. However, intra-patient cycle-to-cycle variability, the lack of standardization in testing methodology, and a limited impact of treatment make NK testing non-beneficial.[17]

Chronic endometritis

CE has been described in the setting of infertility, AUB, and IF.[44] The presence of stromal plasma cells defines CE.[45] However, whether this is a pathologic finding remains unclear.

It has been suggested that the prevalence of CE has been overestimated in the past.[45] This is likely because CE has no clear-cut diagnostic criteria and patients may be entirely asymptomatic.[44,46] In addition, there is no standardization for treatment, and its value has not been firmly established.[44] Diagnostic measures include immunohistochemical (IHC) biopsy staining for CD138 positive plasma cell, tissue culture, and molecular testing for bacterial DNA.[44]

In an attempt to determine if decidual inflammation had long term implications, Goto and colleagues assessed POCs for evidence of chronic deciduitis (CD) and then correlated findings to subsequent pregnancy outcomes. They noted a high rate of CD in both euploid (63.7%) and aneuploid (92%) losses in unexplained RPL patients. CD was also noted in 47% of sporadic losses. However, there were no differences in the subsequent LBR whether or not CD had been noted in the preceding pregnancy.[47]

Kuroda and colleagues observed that CE was almost 6 times more prevalent in infertility patients with endometrial polyps than asymptomatic infertility patients (85.7% vs 15.7% respectively). CE was seen in association with myomas, intrauterine adhesions, and septate uteri as well. Complete resolution of CE was observed via surgery (hysteroscopy) without antibiotic use.[48] Finally, Herlihy and colleagues found that nearly half of 80 IVF patients sampled had greater than 1 CD138 positive cell across 10 high power field (HPF) and that 4% had greater than 10 positive cells per HPF. They found no differences in implantation, clinical pregnancy, clinical pregnancy loss, or LBRs between patients with and without CE.[49] These studies, therefore, raise concerns about testing for CE currently.

Molecular testing of the endometrium

As previously noted, the endometrium is a dynamic epithelium that, in the absence of pregnancy, is continuously cycling between proliferation, differentiation, and destruction. Ovarian steroids drive these transformations. At the simplest level, estrogen drives endometrial proliferation, with progesterone mediating differentiation (**Fig. 1**). As described earlier, endometrial development requires appropriate proliferation which allows for, and is followed by, maturation. It stands to reason that abnormalities in proliferation and/or maturation could impact decidualization. Based on this proliferation/differentiation dyad, most useful markers of endometrial function derive from either of the 2 menstrual cycle phases (**Fig. 2**). It would be presumed as abnormal if an essential marker is absent, excessively expressed, or manifests at an inappropriate time of the cycle.[5]

Regarding unexplained RIF, all markers are suggestive of the same basic issue, an uncoupling of stromal and glandular development. Endometrial glands are sensitive to

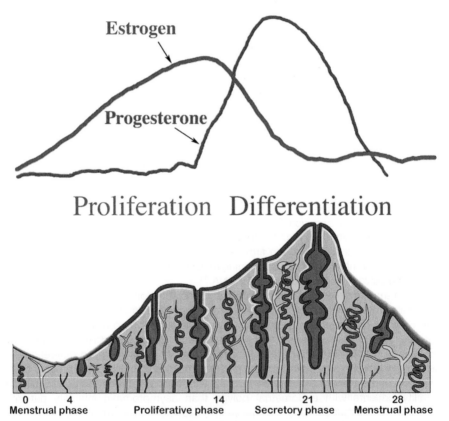

Fig. 1. Endometrial development. Estrogen induces endometrial proliferation, while progesterone blocks proliferation and induces endometrial differentiation.

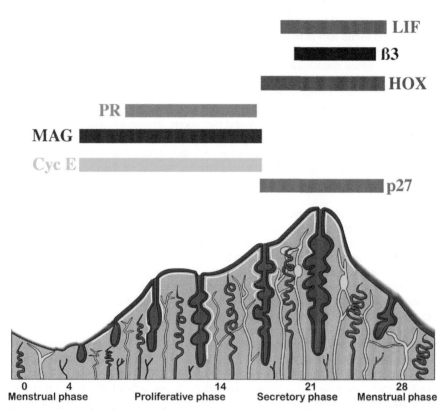

Fig. 2. Markers of endometrial development. Markers of endometrial development (top) logically segregate between the proliferative and differentiation phases of the menstrual cycle (bottom) as the specialized products made in each phase are most often distinct. Cyclin E (Cyc E, the regulator of the Gap 1 to S phase transition of the mitotic cycle); p27 (the specific inhibitor of cyclin E); Mouse Ascites Golgi (MAG; a large mucin found in Blood group A and AB patients); Progesterone receptor (PR, up-regulated by estrogen and down-regulated by progesterone); Homeobox protein HOXA10 (HOX, an endometrial transcription factor); α_v/β_3 integrin (ß3; binding partner of fibronectin); Leukemia inhibitory factor (LIF; promotes cell differentiation).

perturbations during decidualization, especially developmental delay. The endometrial stroma, on the other hand, seems essentially impervious to disruption.[23,50–53] Irrespective of the marker examined, there is a common pattern observed with the stroma matching cycle dating and the glandular development lagging far behind. This pattern has been termed glandular developmental arrest (GDA) and is a marker of delayed endometrial development which Lessey and colleagues described as a Type I implantation defect (where the WOI is delayed[23,52]). Normally the late luteal phase (d24) would demonstrate the absence of progesterone receptor (PR), mouse ascites golgi (MAG), and cyclin E from the endometrial glandular epithelium; while LIF, αv/ß3 integrin (ß3), HOXA10 (HOX), and p27 would be present (see **Fig. 2**). However, in a patient with RIF owing to GDA, MAG, and cyclin E would be present in the glands of the late luteal phase, while LIF, ß3, HOX-A10, and p27 would either be absent or significantly decreased owing to GDA at cycle day 18 to 19.[5] Histologic assessment is insensitive at demonstrating GDA because the Noyes criteria do not reflect the molecular alterations observed with abnormal decidualization.[5]

Molecular testing of the endometrium requires endometrial sampling at a specific time in the cycle. Its aim is to identify potential issues with embryo/endometrial synchrony, errors in endometrial function, or inflammatory factors that may alter endometrial function. While determining the timing of biopsy may seem a simple matter, it depends on whether one considers a natural versus a medicated cycle. Further, numerous cycle preparation regimens exist—i.e., non-agonist, agonist, artificially triggered natural, and progesterone-supplemented natural regimens, to name a few—this can lead to a confusion of terminology and definitions. Therefore, a unifying language to describe the timing of the cycle/biopsy is important. We have presented a key to help simplify the endometrial dating lexicon in **Table 1**. Unification requires aligning identifiable and agreed upon salient events that is, the day of the LH surge, the day of ovulation, embryonic age, or the progesterone start date.

Endometrial receptivity analysis

The endometrial receptivity analysis (ERA) (Igenomix) is the most studied molecular endometrial test. It was designed to date the endometrium by assessing the expression of 238 genes and utilize a machine learning algorithm trained with endometrial histology samples. It aims to "personalize" the timing of the embryo transfer so that the blastocyst would encounter the endometrium at a time normalized to CD 20 which was felt to reflect the optimal WOI.[54] It has been employed to address RIF and enhance the pregnancy likelihood during routine IVF.[44]

The value of the ERA in the setting of RIF has not been established. Ruiz-Alonso and colleagues presented a cohort study employing the ERA in RIF and control subject.[55] They observed similar implantation rates for receptive endometrium (n = 29) and non-receptive/corrected endometria (n = 8) 33.9% and 38.5%, respectively. These implantation rates were less than those reported for those without RIF (n = 11) in their first or second IVF cycle (55%).[55] However, if the cause for RIF was a shift in the WOI, and therefore corrected by the ERA, it should be expected that adjustment would result in a higher implantation rate. In the setting of euploid embryos and RIF, it does not appear that the ERA provides a benefit given that reported LBRs were the same for either standard ET timing or post ERA adjusted ET 50.9% versus 51.6%, respectively.[56]

When focusing on non-RIF IVF patients, the ERA does not appear to be beneficial at improving LBR. Two randomized clinical trials (RCTs) involving good prognosis patients have yielded similar results. Simon and colleagues evaluated the ERA in patients without either RPL or RIF.[57] Their intention to treat analysis demonstrated no significant differences in LBR whether an FET, fresh ET, or ERA-adjusted FET was performed.[57] More recently, Doyle and colleagues reported similar findings following a double blinded RCT involving patients undergoing IVF-PGT-A and ERA. After comparing 381 cycles in which ETs were guided by ERA results to 386 ETs without ERA, these authors noted LBRs of 58.5% and 61.9%, respectively.[58] Cozzolino and colleagues demonstrated worse outcomes for those undergoing autologous or donor IVF cycles in which ERA adjustment was performed.[59] While these results reveal no benefit to the ERA they are consistent with the understanding that the WOI is not a pinpoint. Accordingly, the ERA has begun to fall out of favor[60]

Because the ERA is a molecular means of dating the endometrium and dating abnormalities appear common in fertile women, it should not be surprising that the ERA affords no benefit in the setting of RIF or infertility.[33] It is also not clear why such precise timing would be critical given that the implantation window is at least 3 days long.[3,4] Furthermore, the ERA involves dissolving the biopsy specimen to allow for array testing. As such, it is not possible to perform a histologic assessment of endometrial specimen and therefore, the ERA cannot test for the presence of the pathologic conditions discussed previously (see the endometrial histology section earlier).

Additional array tests built on assessing the WOI include the ER Map, ERPeak, WinTest, and BioER. To date, limited or no published data have emerged, and therefore, their value cannot be assessed.[44,61,62]

ReceptivaDx
The ReceptivaDx evaluates an endometrial sample for the presence of a T helper cell transcription factor serving as a surrogate marker for endometriosis. This makes biologic sense since endometriosis has been shown to influence implantation potential and has a higher prevalence in the infertile population.[63–67] The ReceptivaDX requires endometrial sampling between LH+6 to LH+10 in a natural cycle or P+5 to P+10 in a hormone replacement cycle (see **Table 1**) The ReceptivaDx test does not include a histologic assessment of the biopsied sample, but instead focuses on the IHC expression of B-cell chronic lymphocytic leukemia/lymphoma 6 (BCL6), the aforementioned marker of endometriosis.[68] Almquist and colleagues compared 17 patients with normal BCL6 expression to 52 women with abnormal (increased) BCL6 expression and found a significant decrease in pregnancy and LBRs with increased BCL6 expression.[69] These studies imply that treatment for endometriosis following a positive ReceptivaDx test will improve pregnancy outcomes.[67,70,71] However, in contrast, Klimczak and colleagues recently found that BCL6 expression did not predict live birth in a normal responder IVF population.[72]

Endometrial function test
The Endometrial Function Test (EFT) combines both endometrial histology and an IHC assessment for markers of endometrial development. Histologic examination of P+1 and P+10 endometrial biopsies are assessed for pathologies (acute endometritis, endometrial polyps, etc.) that are known to interfere with endometrial development and implantation.[73] As described earlier, sex steroid changes during the menstrual cycle are responsible for endometrial proliferation followed by differentiation, which includes stromal decidualization (see **Fig. 1**). Although many markers have been proposed to assess these 2 processes, the foundation that all these markers rest upon is the mitotic cycle machinery. This is because cells either proliferate or differentiate—they cannot differentiate until they stop proliferating and differentiated cells do not proliferate. An endometrium that is persistently proliferative cannot generate the cellular factors necessary for blastocyst attachment and implantation. Therefore, the EFT was designed to determine the developmental state of the endometrium by quantitative IHC assessment of a molecular marker of proliferation (cyclin E) and a differentiation marker that stops proliferation (p27)—as described by Dubowy and colleagues[73]

If an endometrial sample from CD 24 still exhibits glandular cyclin E, that is, the glands are still proliferating, then that endometrium cannot be receptive to blastocyst attachment and implantation. Such glands are delayed even though the stroma has reached cycle day 24—the definition of GDA. This is much like a surfer (the glands) who does not engage a wave (the stroma) as it moves past.

By examining a panel of glandular markers on cycle days 15 and 24 the developmental trajectory between these days can be deduced. For example, if a woman's endometrium has developed normally between days 15 and 24, then her endometrium will also be developmentally normal as it passes through the WOI. On the other hand, if her day 15 sample shows too potent a progesterone response and her day 24 biopsy reveals GDA, then adjustments can be made to her protocol to correct these abnormalities. This approach was validated by observing that women who had an abnormal

EFT with no form of intervention were 10.5 times less likely to have an ongoing pregnancy (odds ratio 10.5, 95% CI [confidence interval] 1.29, 680; positive predictive value 1⁄4 91%, 95% CI 72, 100; $P < .001$; Fisher Exact Test) compared to women who had a normal EFT or had an intervention following an abnormal EFT.[74]

The EFT does have limitations. First, 2 biopsies are required for the EFT and processing of the specimens is labor intensive and time consuming. Second, an expert reproductive pathologist is needed to assess the slides produced for the test, and, because the results are the product of human interpretation, read-to-read reliability may limit its validity. However, a cohort of 100 samples were blindly analyzed repeatedly between 3 and 35 times resulting in an excellent intra-observer correlation rating of 0.76 (95% CI 0.70, 0.82).[70,75,76] Given these limitations, use of the EFT should be reserved for cases where there are a small number of embryos available for transfer, such as in cases of donor embryo transfers, transfers after oocyte cryopreservation, or when repletion of embryos is not possible. It should be noted that no RCT assessing the EFT has been performed.[77,78]

Microbiome assessment

The "Colossus of Rhodes" impression of the cervical plug's role in preserving a sterile endometrial state has recently been turned on its head.[79] It appears that few, if any, tissues are truly sterile, with most having a coevolved microbiota. A growing body of evidence supports that the uterus is a low abundance site of bacterial residence with a microbiome projected to be 100 to 10,000 times less populous than the vaginal microbiome.[79]

There is evidence to suggest that an imbalance in the endometrial microbiome, dysbiosis, may be associated with pelvic inflammatory disease, endometriosis, endometrial cancer, infertility, and pregnancy complications.[80] Reports on the ability of the endometrial microbiome to impact implantation grow and suggest that *lactobacillus* dominant (LD) colonization favors implantation.[81,82] However, there remains a challenge in drawing conclusions regarding these emerging data given relatively small study sizes and the potential influence of contamination during trans-cervical endometrial sampling.[79]

Despite such limitations, commercially available tests of the endometrial microbiome are available. Next generation sequencing (NGS) techniques aim to provide a comprehensive assessment of the composition of the endometrial microbiome. The Endometrial Microbiome Metagenomic Analysis (Igenomix) queries an endometrial biopsy for a species-level quantification of the variable microbial 16S rRNA gene via NGS.[83] It then defines the uterine microbiome as either LD (favoring implantation) or non-LD (not favoring implantation). A recent prospective cohort study observed similar cumulative LBRs in those who tested "abnormal" and were treated prior to embryo transfer and those who were not tested prior to emrbyo transfer (36.7% vs 31.2%, respectively).[84]

Presently, there remains no standard for testing the endometrial microbiome, and no clinical trials assessing its role in reproduction have been conducted. More research is needed to best define the optimal make-up of the endometrial microbiome and qualify its role in reproductive health. Therefore, it is important to exert caution when interpreting current data and when considering testing.

CLINICS CARE POINTS

- Endometrial maturation is the process whereby estrogen and progesterone generate a functional epithelium that enables vivo parity.

- During the process of endometrial maturation, the endometrium becomes receptive to an early embryo for a limited time called the window of implantation.
- It is the decidualized endometrium that regulates trophoblastic invasion, prevents uterine rupture, and sets the stage for placentation.
- In the absence of pregnancy, the decidualized endometrium must be discarded and a mature endometrium regenerated in order to reopen the window of implantation.
- Endometrial pathology can lead to abnormal uterine bleeding, cancer, recurrent pregnancy loss, or recurrent implantation failure.
- Testing of the endometrium should be guided based on signs and symptoms.
- Endometrial sampling and histological assessment is helpful in assessing for hyperplasia, carcinoma, retained products of conception, and placental site tumors.
- Dating assessment of the endometrium does not correlate with infertility or recurrent pregnancy loss and screening for a luteal phase defect is no longer advised.
- Ultrasound is helpful in screening assessing endometrial thickness before embryo transfer.
- Molecular testing of the endometrium for recurrent implantation failure, recurrent pregnancy loss, and with assisted reproduction is available, but overall, it has not been demonstrated to improve outcomes.
- The endometrial microbiome may play a role reproductive challenge, however, validated testing and proven treatment benefits remain lacking.
- The widespread implementation novel endometrial diagnostic measures and/or treatments must be evidence based.

DISCLOSURE

The authors have nothing to disclose.

REFERENCES

1. Amoroso EC. The evolution of viviparity. Proc Roy Soc Med 1968;61(11 Pt 2): 1188–200.
2. Kliman HJ. Uteroplacental blood flow. The story of decidualization, menstruation, and trophoblast invasion. Am J Pathol 2000;157(6):1759–68.
3. Navot D, Scott RT, Droesch K, et al. The window of embryo transfer and the efficiency of human conception in vitro. Fertil Steril 1991;55(1):114–8.
4. Wilcox AJ, Baird DD, Weinberg CR. Time of implantation of the conceptus and loss of pregnancy. N Engl J Med 1999;340(23):1796–9.
5. Kliman HJ, Frankfurter D. Clinical approach to recurrent implantation failure: evidence-based evaluation of the endometrium. Fertil Steril 2019;111(4):618–28.
6. van Dijk MM, Kolte AM, Limpens J, et al. Recurrent pregnancy loss: diagnostic workup after two or three pregnancy losses? A systematic review of the literature and meta-analysis. Hum Reprod Update 2020;26(3):356–67.
7. Larsen EC, Christiansen OB, Kolte AM, et al. New insights into mechanisms behind miscarriage. BMC Med 2013;11:154.
8. Busnelli A, Reschini M, Cardellicchio L, et al. How common is real repeated implantation failure? An indirect estimate of the prevalence. Reprod Biomed Online 2020;40(1):91–7.
9. Pirtea P, Cedars MI, Devine K, et al. Recurrent implantation failure: reality or a statistical mirage?: Consensus statement from the July 1, 2022 Lugano Workshop on recurrent implantation failure. Fertil Steril 2023;120(1):45–59.

10. Pirtea P, De Ziegler D, Tao X, et al. Rate of true recurrent implantation failure is low: results of three successive frozen euploid single embryo transfers. Fertil Steril 2021;115(1):45–53.

11. Taylor HS, Pal L, Seli E, et al. Speroff's clinical gynecologic endocrinology and infertility. Ninth edition. Philadelphia: Wolters Kluwer. xiii; 2020. p. 1318.

12. Bergh PA, Navot D. The impact of embryonic development and endometrial maturity on the timing of implantation. Fertil Steril 1992;58(3):537–42.

13. Kliman HJ, Feinberg RF, Haimowitz JE. Human trophoblast-endometrial interactions in an in vitro suspension culture system. Placenta 1990;11(4):349–67.

14. Koelman CA, Coumans AB, Nijman HW, et al. Correlation between oral sex and a low incidence of preeclampsia: a role for soluble HLA in seminal fluid? J Reprod Immunol 2000;46(2):155–66.

15. Ng SW, Norwitz GA, Pavlicev M, et al. Endometrial decidualization: the primary driver of pregnancy health. Int J Mol Sci 2020;21(11).

16. Lessey BA, Damjanovich L, Coutifaris C, et al. Integrin adhesion molecules in the human endometrium. Correlation with the normal and abnormal menstrual cycle. J Clin Invest 1992;90(1):188–95.

17. Polanski LT, Baumgarten M. Endometrial receptivity testing and therapy in assisted reproductive treatment. Semin Reprod Med 2021;39(1–02):27–33.

18. Casarini L, Santi D, Brigante G, et al. Two hormones for one receptor: evolution, biochemistry, actions, and pathophysiology of LH and hCG. Endocr Rev 2018; 39(5):549–92.

19. Macklon NS, Brosens JJ. The human endometrium as a sensor of embryo quality. Biol Reprod 2014;91(4):98.

20. Dey SK, Lim H, Das SK, et al. Molecular cues to implantation. Endocr Rev 2004; 25(3):341–73.

21. Brosens JJ, Salker MS, Teklenburg G, et al. Uterine selection of human embryos at implantation. Sci Rep 2014;4:3894.

22. Schwenke M, Knöfler M, Velicky P, et al. Control of human endometrial stromal cell motility by PDGF-BB, HB-EGF and trophoblast-secreted factors. PLoS One 2013;8(1):e54336.

23. Lessey BA, Castelbaum AJ, Sawin SW, et al. Integrins as markers of uterine receptivity in women with primary unexplained infertility. Fertil Steril 1995;63(3): 535–42.

24. Neal SA, Morin SJ, Franasiak JM, et al. Preimplantation genetic testing for aneuploidy is cost-effective, shortens treatment time, and reduces the risk of failed embryo transfer and clinical miscarriage. Fertil Steril 2018;110(5):896–904.

25. Wentz AC, Herbert CM, Maxson WS, et al. Cycle of conception endometrial biopsy. Fertil Steril 1986;46(2):196–9.

26. Holden EC, Kashani BN, Morelli SS, et al. Improved outcomes after blastocyst-stage frozen-thawed embryo transfers compared with cleavage stage: a society for assisted reproductive technologies clinical outcomes reporting system study. Fertil Steril 2018;110(1):89–94 e2.

27. CDC. Assisted reproductive technology National summary report. US Dept of Health and Human Services; 2017.

28. Munro MG, Critchley HOD, Broder MS, et al. FIGO classification system (PALM-COEIN) for causes of abnormal uterine bleeding in nongravid women of reproductive age. Int J Gynaecol Obstet 2011;113(1):3–13.

29. Garneau AS, Young SL. Defining recurrent implantation failure: a profusion of confusion or simply an illusion? Fertil Steril 2021;116(6):1432–5.

30. Ata B, Kalafat E, Somigliana E. A new definition of recurrent implantation failure on the basis of anticipated blastocyst aneuploidy rates across female age. Fertil Steril 2021;116(5):1320–7.

31. Noyes RW, Hertig AT, Rock J. Reprint of: dating the endometrial biopsy. Fertil Steril 2019;112(4 Suppl1):e93–115.

32. Practice Committee of the American Society for Reproductive M. Current clinical irrelevance of luteal phase deficiency: a committee opinion. Fertil Steril 2015; 103(4):e27–32.

33. Coutifaris C, Myers ER, Guzick DS, et al. Histological dating of timed endometrial biopsy tissue is not related to fertility status. Fertil Steril 2004;82(5):1264–72.

34. Perez-Medina T, Bajo-Arenas J, Salazar F, et al. Endometrial polyps and their implication in the pregnancy rates of patients undergoing intrauterine insemination: a prospective, randomized study. Hum Reprod 2005;20(6):1632–5.

35. Kitaya K, Takeuchi T, Mizuta S, et al. Endometritis: new time, new concepts. Fertil Steril 2018;110(3):344–50.

36. Craciunas L, Gallos I, Chu J, et al. Conventional and modern markers of endometrial receptivity: a systematic review and meta-analysis. Hum Reprod Update 2019;25(2):202–23.

37. Gao G, Cui X, Li S, et al. Endometrial thickness and IVF cycle outcomes: a meta-analysis. Reprod Biomed Online 2020;40(1):124–33.

38. Liu KE, Hartman M, Hartman A, et al. The impact of a thin endometrial lining on fresh and frozen-thaw IVF outcomes: an analysis of over 40 000 embryo transfers. Hum Reprod 2018;33(10):1883–8.

39. Mahutte N, Hartman M, Meng L, et al. Optimal endometrial thickness in fresh and frozen-thaw in vitro fertilization cycles: an analysis of live birth rates from 96,000 autologous embryo transfers. Fertil Steril 2022;117(4):792–800.

40. Zhang J, Liu H, Mao X, et al. Effect of endometrial thickness on birthweight in frozen embryo transfer cycles: an analysis including 6181 singleton newborns. Hum Reprod 2019;34(9):1707–15.

41. Ayida G, Chamberlain P, Barlow D, et al. Uterine cavity assessment prior to in vitro fertilization: comparison of transvaginal scanning, saline contrast hysterosonography and hysteroscopy. Ultrasound Obstet Gynecol 1997;10(1):59–62.

42. Varasteh NN, Neuwirth RS, Levin B, et al. Pregnancy rates after hysteroscopic polypectomy and myomectomy in infertile women. Obstet Gynecol 1999;94(2): 168–71.

43. Pritts EA, Parker WH, Olive DL. Fibroids and infertility: an updated systematic review of the evidence. Fertil Steril 2009;91(4):1215–23.

44. Clain EDK, Devine K. Endometrial receptivity, to test or not to test: the evidence on contemporary assays. Fertility and Sterility Reviews 2023;4(1):50–65.

45. Liu Y, Chen X, Huang J, et al. Comparison of the prevalence of chronic endometritis as determined by means of different diagnostic methods in women with and without reproductive failure. Fertil Steril 2018;109(5):832–9.

46. Greenwood SM, Moran JJ. Chronic endometritis: morphologic and clinical observations. Obstet Gynecol 1981;58(2):176–84.

47. Goto T, Goto S, Ozawa F, et al. The association between chronic deciduitis and recurrent pregnancy loss. J Reprod Immunol 2023;156:103824.

48. Kuroda K, Yamanaka A, Takamizawa S, et al. Prevalence of and risk factors for chronic endometritis in patients with intrauterine disorders after hysteroscopic surgery. Fertil Steril 2022;118(3):568–75.

49. Herlihy NS, Klimczak AM, Titus S, et al. The role of endometrial staining for CD138 as a marker of chronic endometritis in predicting live birth. J Assist Reprod Genet 2022;39(2):473–9.

50. Bonhoff A, Johannisson E, Bohnet HG. Morphometric analysis of the endometrium of infertile patients in relation to peripheral hormone levels. Fertil Steril 1990;54(1):84–9.

51. Benadiva CA, Metzger DA. Superovulation with human menopausal gonadotropins is associated with endometrial gland-stroma dyssynchrony. Fertil Steril 1994;61(4):700–4.

52. Kliman HJ FR, Vandeerlin P, Barmat LI, et al. Glandular developmental arrest (GDA): a unifying model of reproductive endometrial pathology. Fertil Steril 1997;68:S96–7.

53. Basir GS, O WS, Ng EH, et al. Morphometric analysis of peri-implantation endometrium in patients having excessively high oestradiol concentrations after ovarian stimulation. Hum Reprod 2001;16(3):435–40.

54. Valdes CT, Schutt A, Simon C. Implantation failure of endometrial origin: it is not pathology, but our failure to synchronize the developing embryo with a receptive endometrium. Fertil Steril 2017;108(1):15–8.

55. Ruiz-Alonso M, Blesa D, Díaz-Gimeno P, et al. The endometrial receptivity array for diagnosis and personalized embryo transfer as a treatment for patients with repeated implantation failure. Fertil Steril 2013;100(3):818–24.

56. Tan J, Kan A, Hitkari J, et al. The role of the endometrial receptivity array (ERA) in patients who have failed euploid embryo transfers. J Assist Reprod Genet 2018; 35(4):683–92.

57. Simon C, Gómez C, Cabanillas S, et al. A 5-year multicentre randomized controlled trial comparing personalized, frozen and fresh blastocyst transfer in IVF. Reprod Biomed Online 2020;41(3):402–15.

58. Doyle N, Jahandideh S, Hill MJ, et al. Effect of timing by endometrial receptivity testing vs standard timing of frozen embryo transfer on live birth in patients undergoing in vitro fertilization: a randomized clinical trial. JAMA 2022;328(21): 2117–25.

59. Cozzolino M, Diáz-Gimeno P, Pellicer A, et al. Use of the endometrial receptivity array to guide personalized embryo transfer after a failed transfer attempt was associated with a lower cumulative and per transfer live birth rate during donor and autologous cycles. Fertil Steril 2022;118(4):724–36.

60. Raff M, Jacobs E, Voorhis BV. End of an endometrial receptivity array? Fertil Steril 2022;118(4):737.

61. Enciso M, Carrascosa JP, Sarasa J, et al. Development of a new comprehensive and reliable endometrial receptivity map (ER Map/ER Grade) based on RT-qPCR gene expression analysis. Hum Reprod 2018;33(2):220–8.

62. Suhorutshenko M, Kukushkina V, Velthut-Meikas A, et al. Endometrial receptivity revisited: endometrial transcriptome adjusted for tissue cellular heterogeneity. Hum Reprod 2018;33(11):2074–86.

63. Ryan IP, Taylor RN. Endometriosis and infertility: new concepts. Obstet Gynecol Surv 1997;52(6):365–71.

64. Kao LC, Germeyer A, Tulac S, et al. Expression profiling of endometrium from women with endometriosis reveals candidate genes for disease-based implantation failure and infertility. Endocrinology 2003;144(7):2870–81.

65. Pritts EA, Taylor RN. An evidence-based evaluation of endometriosis-associated infertility. Endocrinol Metab Clin N Am 2003;32(3):653–67.

66. Zanatta A, Rocha AM, Carvalho FM, et al. The role of the Hoxa10/HOXA10 gene in the etiology of endometriosis and its related infertility: a review. J Assist Reprod Genet 2010;27(12):701–10.

67. Isono W, Wada-Hiraike O, Akino N, et al. The efficacy of non-assisted reproductive technology treatment might be limited in infertile patients with advanced endometriosis in their 30s. J Obstet Gynaecol Res 2019;45(2):368–75.

68. Evans-Hoeker E, Lessey BA, Jeong JW, et al. Endometrial BCL6 Overexpression in Eutopic Endometrium of Women With Endometriosis. Reprod Sci 2016;23(9): 1234–41.

69. Almquist LD, Likes CE, Stone B, et al. Endometrial BCL6 testing for the prediction of in vitro fertilization outcomes: a cohort study. Fertil Steril 2017;108(6): 1063–9.

70. Macer ML, Taylor HS. Endometriosis and infertility: a review of the pathogenesis and treatment of endometriosis-associated infertility. Obstet Gynecol Clin N Am 2012;39(4):535–49.

71. Soriano D, Adler I, Bouaziz J, et al. Fertility outcome of laparoscopic treatment in patients with severe endometriosis and repeated in vitro fertilization failures. Fertil Steril 2016;106(5):1264–9.

72. Klimczak AM, Herlihy NS, Scott CS, et al. B-cell lymphoma 6 expression is not associated with live birth in a normal responder in vitro fertilization population. Fertil Steril 2022;117(2):351–8.

73. Dubowy RL, Feinberg RF, Keefe DL, et al. Improved endometrial assessment using cyclin E and p27. Fertil Steril 2003;80(1):146–56.

74. Kliman HJ MJ, Grunert GM, Cardone VRS, et al. The endometrial function test (EFT) directs care and predicts ART outcome. Fertil Steril 2002;78:S17.

75. Cicchetti DV. Multiple comparison methods: establishing guidelines for their valid application in neuropsychological research. J Clin Exp Neuropsychol 1994;16(1): 155–61.

76. Stephenson MD, McQueen D, Winter M, et al. Luteal start vaginal micronized progesterone improves pregnancy success in women with recurrent pregnancy loss. Fertil Steril 2017;107(3):684–690 e2.

77. Kliman HJ, Honig S, Walls D, et al. Optimization of endometrial preparation results in a normal endometrial function test (EFT) and good reproductive outcome in donor ovum recipients. J Assist Reprod Genet 2006;23(7–8):299–303.

78. Crawford S, Boulet SL, Kawwass JF, et al. Cryopreserved oocyte versus fresh oocyte assisted reproductive technology cycles, United States, 2013. Fertil Steril 2017;107(1):110–8.

79. Baker JM, Chase DM, Herbst-Kralovetz MM. Uterine microbiota: residents, tourists, or invaders? Front Immunol 2018;9:208.

80. Molina NM, Sola-Leyva A, Haahr T, et al. Analysing endometrial microbiome: methodological considerations and recommendations for good practice. Hum Reprod 2021;36(4):859–79.

81. Moreno I, Codoñer FM, Vilella F, et al. Evidence that the endometrial microbiota has an effect on implantation success or failure. Am J Obstet Gynecol 2016; 215(6):684–703.

82. Franasiak JM, Scott RT Jr. Recurrent implantation failure : etiologies and clinical management. In: Microbiome in embryonic implantation and implantation failure. Cham: Springer International Publishing : Imprint: Springer; 2018. p. 1, online resource (XIII, 215 pages 32 illustrations, 29 illustrations in color.

83. Franasiak JM, Werner MD, Juneau CR, et al. Endometrial microbiome at the time of embryo transfer: next-generation sequencing of the 16S ribosomal subunit. J Assist Reprod Genet 2016;33(1):129–36.
84. Iwami N, Kawamata M, Ozawa N, et al. Therapeutic intervention based on gene sequencing analysis of microbial 16S ribosomal RNA of the intrauterine microbiome improves pregnancy outcomes in IVF patients: a prospective cohort study. J Assist Reprod Genet 2023;40(1):125–35.

Contemporary Management of the Patient with Polycystic Ovary Syndrome

Nicolás Omar Francone, MD[a,b], Tia Ramirez, MD[a,b],
Christina E. Boots, MD, MSCI[b,*]

KEYWORDS

- Polycystic ovary syndrome • Infertility • Fertility • Lifestyle • Ovulation

KEY POINTS

- Polycystic ovary syndrome (PCOS) is a complex syndrome requiring a multidisciplinary approach to care.
- The PCOS phenotype is diverse, and thus, treatment should be individualized.
- All individuals with PCOS should receive counseling around the 5 tenets of PCOS:
  - Menstrual cyclicity and endometrial protection.
  - Hyperandrogenism.
  - Metabolic health.
  - Mental health.
  - Current or future fertility.

INTRODUCTION

Polycystic ovary syndrome (PCOS) is one of the most common reproductive disorders, affecting approximately 10% of women. The most used criteria for the clinical diagnosis were established in 2003 in Rotterdam and include 2 of 3 symptoms: oligo-ovulation or anovulation, clinical or biochemical signs of hyperandrogenism, and polycystic ovaries on ultrasound. However, defining each of these criteria can be difficult and many individuals struggle for years to confirm the diagnosis of PCOS. In addition to the variability of the reproductive features of this disorder, the Rotterdam criteria (and others) fail to include the metabolic aspects that are so often associated with the diagnosis. Metabolic features present in many individuals with PCOS include difficulty with weight management, insulin resistance, dyslipidemia, nonalcoholic fatty liver disease, disordered sleep breathing, and increased risk of

[a] McGaw Medical Center of Northwestern University; [b] Division of Reproductive Endocrinology and Infertility, 259 East Erie, Suite 2400, Chicago, IL 60611, USA
* Corresponding author.
E-mail address: christina.boots@nm.org

Obstet Gynecol Clin N Am 50 (2023) 695–705
https://doi.org/10.1016/j.ogc.2023.08.003
0889-8545/23/© 2023 Elsevier Inc. All rights reserved.
obgyn.theclinics.com

long-term cardiovascular dysfunction. The combination of both a dysfunctional reproductive axis as well as metabolic disturbances also increases the risk for infertility and mental health disorders.

In this review of the clinical management of PCOS, we will summarize the diagnostic criteria and the management options for each of these symptoms. It is critical to note that no 2 individuals will have the same presentation, nor will their symptoms and concerns remain the same throughout their reproductive life. As described by Dr Fritz in *Clinical Gynecologic Endocrinology and Infertility*, *"the primary advantage to having specific diagnostic criteria for PCOS relates to research, because varying criteria cloud the conclusions and questions the generalizability of results from studies involving women with 'PCOS'. In clinical medicine, simply knowing & understanding the health implications & consequences of chronic anovulation and methods for their effective management are far more important than assigning a specific diagnosis of PCOS..."*[1] Clinical care for PCOS should be individualized for each patient and should focus on the symptoms that concern them, as well as the opportunity for prevention of long-term consequences. This care should be comprehensive, creative, and thoughtful to address all aspects of PCOS. Often, this can best, and perhaps only, be done with a multidisciplinary approach. Dedicated PCOS clinics now exist and have effectively treated these individuals. However, gynecologists and reproductive endocrinologists can be the primary managers of PCOS when combined with a network of experienced, empathic providers that specialize in dermatology, mental health, nutrition, obesity, endocrinology, primary care, and so forth.

When we care for individuals with PCOS, our goal should be to clarify the diagnosis of PCOS and educate our patients about what this condition means for their current, short-term, and long-term health. This review will address each aspect of PCOS by organizing the discussion by systems: menstrual cycles and endometrial protection, hyperandrogenism, metabolic dysfunction, mental health and, finally, infertility (**Fig. 1**).

ENDOMETRIAL PROTECTION AND MENSTRUAL CYCLICITY

PCOS is linked to chronic anovulation and irregular menstrual cycles. Oligomenorrhea is defined as cycles occurring less frequently than every 35 days, or fewer than 8 cycles per year.[2] Increasingly, individuals recognize menstrual cyclicity as a vital sign of good health and oligomenorrhea, amenorrhea, or dysfunctional uterine bleeding can be distressing and contribute to a poor quality of life. This distress is in addition to the risks of endometrial hyperplasia and cancer associated with prolonged unopposed exposure of the endometrium to estradiol. Educating patients about the

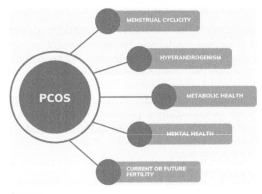

Fig. 1. Five tenets of PCOS.

hypothalamic-pituitary dysfunction that results from PCOS is important as we help them understand the potential mechanisms for therapy. Individuals are often frustrated by an unexplained prescription for birth control pills. However, the better they understand the mechanism by which progestins (± estradiol) improve their cycles and protect their endometrium, the more empowered they are to utilize these therapies effectively. Combined ethinyl estradiol + progestin pills/patches/rings, progestin-only pills, depot progesterone, progesterone implants as well as levonorgestrel intrauterine devices (IUDs) are commonly used to regulate menstrual cycles and improve symptoms in women with PCOS. Combined ethinyl estradiol-progestin oral pills have been shown to effectively regulate menstrual cycles in women with PCOS. A systematic review and meta-analysis of 16 randomized controlled trials (RCTs) found that the combination pill significantly increased the frequency of menstrual cycles in women with PCOS compared to placebo or no treatment.[3] IUDs containing levonorgestrel have also been shown to effectively regulate menstrual cycles in women with PCOS and decrease endometrial proliferation.[4] Patients should be involved in the decision regarding which medication is right for them and when to initiate said medication.

While hormonal therapy is the gold standard for managing symptoms of oligomenorrhea, amenorrhea, and dysfunctional uterine bleeding, lifestyle changes and improved insulin sensitivity can also improve menstrual regularity. In the classic Pregnancy in Polycystic Ovary Syndrome I (PPCOS1) trial, metformin achieved ovulatory cycles in 29% of women. While this study proved that clomiphene citrate was superior for ovulation induction, it clearly also demonstrates that in some women, metformin alone is an option. This is particularly useful in women with a poor tolerance or contraindication to hormonal therapy.[5]

HYPERANDROGENISM

Hyperandrogenism is a hallmark sign of PCOS and is often what leads patients to seek care. It manifests as acne, hirsutism, or alopecia, which can be quite bothersome for patients. Its presentation ranges from mild to severe and tends to be more insidious than acute in onset. Approximately 75% to 80% of patients presenting with features of hyperandrogenism will have PCOS. It is exceedingly rare for patients with PCOS to present with virilization, and in such cases, a full workup must be performed to rule out other etiologies such as androgen-secreting tumors.

The evaluation for patients presenting with hyperandrogenism includes serum laboratory evaluation as well as a physical examination. Current recommendations include obtaining total serum testosterone and morning, follicular phase 17-hydroxyprogesterone (17OHP) levels in all patients presenting with hyperandrogenism in the setting of oligomenorrhea.[6] Although it is the unbound serum testosterone that ultimately causes hyperandrogenic symptoms, it is not necessary to evaluate free testosterone given the unreliability of testing assays. If total testosterone is elevated, it can be assumed that there is also an elevation of free testosterone. Severely elevated testosterone levels should prompt thorough evaluation of other causes, such as ovarian and adrenal tumors. 17OHP is obtained to exclude nonclassical congenital adrenal hyperplasia (NCCAH) given its similar presentation to PCOS. Populations at higher risk of NCCAH are Eastern European Jews and women of Hispanic, Slavic, or Italian descent.[7] There appears to be a role in obtaining androstenedione levels in certain populations; however, this relationship has not been fully elucidated, and should only be ordered with a high clinical suspicion of PCOS in the setting of normal serum testosterone levels.[8]

The persistent elevation of androgens in people with PCOS affects the synthesis of multiple proteins, particularly a decrease in the amount of sex hormone–binding globulin (SHBG). Lower levels of SHBG allow for higher levels of free testosterone which disrupt ovarian theca cell function, further exacerbating the cycle of anovulation, and directly causing symptoms of clinical hyperandrogenism. When the patient's primary goal in the treatment of PCOS is not fertility, then the best mechanism to decrease serum testosterone is via pituitary suppression. The gold-standard suppression remains combined oral estradiol and progestin therapy. Any systemic progestins ± estradiol therapy will suppress both follicle stimulating hormone (FSH) and luteinizing hormone (LH). This reduction in LH removes stimulation to the theca cells and thus lowers serum androgens. Oral estradiol has the added benefit of increasing hepatic production of SHBG and thus further decreasing free testosterone.

Given hormonal therapy may be undesirable or contraindicated in some patients, alternative treatments have been studied for the treatment of hyperandrogenism. Spironolactone, a mineralocorticoid inhibitor, has been shown to be effective at reducing the symptoms of hyperandrogenism, particularly acne. In our practice, we rarely venture into additional agents such as 5-alpha reductase inhibitors, given the increased risks and side effect profiles. Lifestyle improvements that result in improved insulin and glucose sensitivity may also provide beneficial outcomes. Circulating insulin stimulates insulin-like growth factor receptors prompting the ovary to synthesize additional testosterone. Thus, decreased insulin should modestly improve ovarian androgen production and possibly clinical hyperandrogenism. Metformin and other insulin sensitizing agents may provide similar benefits.

It is important to set expectations for results with patients. Many features of hyperandrogenism are not completely reversible. When a vellus hair becomes a terminal hair, it never reverts back. Rather, hormonal therapy will only help to decrease the rate of terminal hair conversion. Co-management with dermatology specialists should always be considered. Topical and cosmetic therapies are often recommended in addition to hormonal therapy to achieve optimal cosmetic results. Many of these can be used during fertility treatment and include topical eflornithine, waxing, and laser hair removal.

METABOLIC DYSFUNCTION

PCOS is linked to multiple metabolic abnormalities including obesity, insulin resistance and diabetes, cardiovascular dysfunction, nonalcoholic fatty liver disease, and disordered sleep breathing. Screening for these conditions should be performed at annual primary care and gynecologic visits as well as preconception.

There is a complex interaction between obesity and PCOS. Numerous studies have demonstrated an elevated risk and earlier onset of being overweight/obese in people with PCOS. This resultant increase in body mass index (BMI), and possibly associated unhealthy lifestyle, further exacerbates both the metabolic and reproductive phenotypes associated with PCOS. However, there are limited studies using an unselected population, meaning that individuals are screened in the community rather than limiting the pool of individuals with PCOS to those who present for clinical care, thereby biasing the studies toward worse phenotypes. In these unselected studies, individuals with PCOS have similar BMI to women without PCOS, and there is a nearly uniform prevalence worldwide, despite varying prevalence of obesity. While obesity may serve as a driver for referral, it does not appear to be a direct cause of PCOS development. Nonetheless, obesity remains an independent and additive risk factor for metabolic disease in individuals with PCOS.[9–12]

Regardless of BMI, women with PCOS have adipose tissue dysfunction and altered distribution. With increased abdominal/visceral fat distribution, the adipocytes are often larger, have lower lipase activity, impaired lipolysis, and favor insulin resistance and subclinical inflammation.[13,14]

Given the high prevalence of insulin resistance and hyperinsulinemia in PCOS, all patients should be screened with either a 2-hour oral glucose tolerance test (OGTT) or a fasting glucose with hemoglobin A1C measurement. Individuals with normal OGTTs should be rescreened every 2 years whereas people with abnormal OGTTs should be rescreened annually for the development of diabetes. Hyperinsulinemia is known to exacerbate hyperandrogenism by both stimulating production of androgens and decreasing the production of SHBG, further demanding the need for effective treatment options. Regardless of laboratory diagnosis of insulin resistance, prediabetes, or diabetes, it is important to counsel all individuals with PCOS regarding the adoption of a healthy lifestyle. Given that there is likely already cellular dysfunction in glucose metabolism, particularly in adipocytes, lifestyle interventions may play a crucial role in halting the progression to overt glucose intolerance.

Lifestyle modification with diet, exercise, and behavioral change has been shown to be the most effective intervention to improve obesity, insulin resistance, and cardiovascular outcomes.[15] Modest reductions in weight (5%–10%) lead to significant improvement in these 3 factors in part due to improved lipid profile, specifically total and low-density lipoprotein cholesterol, and decreased adipose tissue.[15,16] While specific exercise recommendations do not exist for this population, aerobic exercise multiple times per week has been shown to reduce insulin resistance and obesity and improve lipid profiles if performed consistently over more than 12 weeks.[17] All patients, regardless of their BMI, should be asked about barriers to physical activity and counseled appropriately. We should encourage our patients to incorporate diverse physical activities into their daily life for both metabolic and mental health benefits.

Nutritional patterns should model the Mediterranean diet, which is well-known to improve cardiovascular dysfunction. The Mediterranean pattern of eating focuses on vegetables and fruits, proteins from plants, fish or lean meats, healthy fats, moderating complex carbohydrates, and minimizing simple sugars. Much like co-managing hyperandrogenism with dermatology colleagues, there is a great opportunity to involve nutritionists and dieticians in the management of patients with PCOS. Thus, nutritional recommendations will be enhanced and individualized by an experienced and empathetic registered dietician.

Making these lifestyle modifications without experiencing any weight loss still has health benefits. Good health at most BMI levels can be achieved and we should discuss this with our patients. However, the desire for weight loss should be addressed and a referral to physicians who specialize in obesity medicine should be made. Lifestyle and obesity specialists have the experience as well as the clinical support to provide comprehensive weight loss care that would include nutrition consults, psychological support, as well as access to weight loss medications and/or surgery.

In addition to lifestyle modifications, there is growing evidence for the use of insulin sensitizing agents in individuals with PCOS. Metformin is the most well studied and demonstrates effective diabetes prevention as well as improved menstrual cycles, hyperandrogenism, and BMI when used in combination with lifestyle modifications.[16,18] Glucagon-like peptide 1 (GLP-1) analogs are being studied in populations of obese patients with PCOS and have preliminarily shown promising results in both improving insulin resistance and hyperandrogenism and promoting weight loss.[19]

Finally, integrative medicine can be beneficial in metabolic health as well. The dietary supplement myo-inositol has been studied as a means to improve insulin sensitivity and possibly improve oligomenorrhea.[20] Herbal therapy has also shown benefits when provided by experienced Chinese medicine practitioners. Lastly, evidence extrapolated from the general cardiovascular literature would suggest that vitamin D and omega 3 fatty acid supplements may also benefit individuals with PCOS.

MENTAL HEALTH RISKS AND INTERVENTIONS

PCOS is associated with an increased risk of depression, anxiety, disordered eating, and poor body image. Several studies have shown a high prevalence of moderate to severe depressive and anxiety symptoms in women with PCOS, with a systematic review and meta-analysis reporting an increased risk for abnormal depression scores in these individuals.[19–22] These mental health concerns are also independently associated with obesity and diabetes, thus those individuals with both PCOS and bigger bodies carry even higher risks. Additionally, individuals with PCOS are at a higher risk of developing disordered eating behaviors and body image concerns due to symptoms such as weight gain, hirsutism, and acne.[23–25] These issues can significantly affect the quality of life, highlighting the importance of acknowledging and treating them. Several interventions have been shown to be effective in improving depression, anxiety, and body image problems in PCOS patients, including medication and cognitive-behavioral therapy.[26,27] Therefore, educating individuals of these risks, early identification, and referral to caring and empathetic mental health providers for treatment of these issues can improve the overall well-being of women with PCOS.

FERTILITY

Women with PCOS have higher rates of infertility. Delayed conception is mostly due to oligo-ovulation or anovulation, with additive influence from metabolic dysfunction, specifically insulin resistance. Women with PCOS should be educated and counseled about the higher risk of infertility. However, reassurance should also be provided that most PCOS-associated infertility has a relatively simple and effective treatment option. Comprehensive counseling when the PCOS diagnosis is made should clearly explain the fertility physiology, review opportunities to lower the risk of anovulation and infertility, and discuss the treatment options available. All individuals with PCOS should be recommended to schedule a preconception consult prior to trying to conceive as this creates an opportunity to screen for metabolic and thyroid dysfunction, counsel on pregnancy-specific nutrition and activity, and make a fertility game plan. Suppose individuals experience oligo-ovulation or anovulation for 60 days or more after stopping contraception. In that case, it may be beneficial to schedule a follow-up visit promptly to discuss potential ovulation induction therapy and a thorough fertility evaluation.

When any woman presents with delayed conception and/or a diagnosis of infertility, several factors should be considered from the start: (1) preconception testing and counseling, (2) maternal age and family-building goals, and (3) other infertility risk factors.

The workup for infertility in patients with PCOS typically begins with a detailed medical history and physical examination. In addition, initial laboratory testing should include the standard of care preconception evaluation, which includes complete blood count, liver and kidney function tests, fasting glucose and insulin levels, lipid profile, and thyroid-stimulating hormone level. Other etiologies such as tubal factor or uterine factor infertility should be ruled out with either a saline-infused sonogram or hysterosalpingogram. Additionally, male factor infertility must also be ruled out with history, physical examination, and semen analysis. A secondary analysis of the PPCOS trial showed that at least 4% of women presenting with anovulatory PCOS infertility also had bilateral tubal occlusion and another 10+% had concomitant oligospermia.[28] This suggests that while all of these women had ovulatory dysfunction, not all of them were purely anovulatory, and in these cases where women with PCOS at least intermittently cycled, a thorough evaluation for other contributing causes of infertility should be considered. Once the workup is complete, the results can help guide treatment decisions and identify any potential obstacles to achieving a successful pregnancy.

Lifestyle Modifications

One of the first-line treatments for infertility in patients with PCOS is lifestyle modification, including nutrition, physical activity, and possibly weight loss. An assessment of their current lifestyle habits should be performed and incorporated into a conversation about whether improvements can be made while pursuing conception and fertility treatment. Some individuals desire and benefit from time focused on these modifications prior to conception. While weight loss resulting from caloric deficit or medications may be harmful to early pregnancy, adopting healthy dietary patterns and exercise habits during the active conception phase can be beneficial. The decision regarding whether to pursue treatment immediately versus focused lifestyle modifications needs to be considered with maternal age, maternal BMI, other comorbidities, and the patient's preferences. As mentioned in the *Metabolic Dysfunction* section, nutrition referrals as well as medications, specifically metformin and GLP-1 agonists, may be beneficial. Current recommendations are to discontinue GLP-1 agonists at least 1 to 2 months prior to conception, depending on the half-life.[29] It is also important to note that many women with PCOS suffer or have suffered from disordered eating, and thus overemphasis on weight loss can be triggering. Screening for disordered eating and ensuring they have appropriate mental health support is an important component in lifestyle counseling.

There are limited data on the benefit of focused lifestyle improvements prior to fertility treatment. The OWL PCOS (Treatment of Hyperandrogenism Versus Insulin Resistance in Infertile Polycystic Ovary Syndrome Women) study was a 2-site RCT that randomized 149 women with PCOS to 1 of 3 arms: oral contraceptive pills (OCPs) only, lifestyle modifications alone, or both, prior to fertility treatment. The lifestyle modification arm included caloric restriction, increased physical activity, behavioral modification, and weight loss medications. The lifestyle arm had significantly more weight loss than the OCP arm, although the dropout rate was ~13%. Women in the lifestyle arm were more likely to ovulate, but there was no statistical improvement in pregnancy, miscarriage, or live birth.[30] Individualized assessment regarding delayed conception for lifestyle modifications should be done with each woman, especially given the sparse data on benefits, modest weight loss, and high dropout rates. Nonetheless, healthy nutrition and improved quality and quantity of physical activity should be encouraged.

Oral Ovulation Induction

The first-line treatment for infertility in patients with PCOS is typically oral ovulation induction agents, such as clomiphene citrate or letrozole. Clomiphene citrate is a selective estrogen receptor modulator (SERM) that works by inhibiting negative feedback of estrogen at the hypothalamus, resulting in an increase in FSH secretion with subsequent follicular growth and ovulation. Letrozole, an aromatase inhibitor (AI), works by inhibiting the conversion of androgens to estrogen, resulting in a decrease in negative feedback at the hypothalamus and subsequent increase in FSH secretion. Studies comparing clomiphene citrate and letrozole in treating infertility in patients with PCOS have yielded mixed results, though evidence shows a likely increased ovulation and birth rate with letrozole as a first-line treatment. The PPCOSII RCT of 750 infertile women with PCOS found that letrozole was more effective than clomiphene citrate in inducing ovulation (61.7% vs 48.3%) and achieving live births (27.5% vs 19.1%);[31] however, a systematic review and meta-analysis of 21 RCTs involving 3235 women with PCOS found no significant difference in live birth rates between the 2 medications.[32] Interestingly, the benefit of letrozole over clomiphene citrate was heightened in individuals of an elevated BMI, whereas there was no difference in those with a normal BMI. In women resistant to either clomiphene alone or letrozole alone, there are data to suggest improved ovulation when the 2 medications are taken together.[33] Patients should be counseled that unlike clomiphene citrate, the use of letrozole for ovulation induction is off-label, with many studies showing its efficacy and safety.

When starting oral ovulation induction, women may benefit from an initial progestin withdrawal bleed if they have prolonged amenorrhea. The starting dose should consider the number of missed ovulatory cycles and maternal age, but typically, it is recommended to start with the lowest effective dose. If there is no response to the initial dose as noted via ovulation predictor kits, absence of a period, or ultrasound and laboratory monitoring, the dose can be immediately increased and repeated without requiring an additional progestin withdrawal bleed.

Metformin is often used alone or in addition to ovulation induction agents. The original PPCOS1 trial showed that clomiphene was superior to metformin alone. However, there was no difference in live birth rates between clomiphene alone versus clomiphene plus metformin. There is currently limited evidence on the use of metformin in addition to ovulation induction with clomiphene citrate or letrozole for patients with PCOS who do not have insulin resistance. Other insulin sensitizers have been studied and may increase ovulation rates in patients with PCOS, particularly recent and ongoing studies using GLP-1 agonists.[29,34]

Exogenous Gonadotropins

When patients do not respond to lifestyle modifications or oral ovulation induction with SERMs or AIs, exogenous gonadotropins may be considered as a treatment option. It is important to note that the use of gonadotropins is associated with a significantly higher risk of a multiple gestation pregnancy. As a result, thorough counseling and a low-dose regimen should be utilized to minimize these risks. To prevent confusion between baseline cysts and developing follicles, it is recommended to conduct a baseline ultrasound prior to initiating ovulation induction with gonadotropins. Subsequently, transvaginal ultrasounds should be performed to monitor the quantity and size of growing follicles as well as endometrial thickness. Current research comparing gonadotropin regimens in this patient population has not yielded a definitive advantage for either FSH alone or a combination of FSH with LH.

In Vitro Fertilization

In vitro fertilization (IVF) should be considered when oral therapy has either failed to induce ovulation or if several cycles of ovulation have failed to achieve a pregnancy. When to transition from oral therapy to IVF depends on many factors including the financial burden and insurance coverage, its effects on mental health and burnout, and the impact of other etiologies of infertility such as tubal or male factor. Additionally, maternal age and family-building goals should be considered when deciding when to pursue IVF as embryo cryopreservation has benefits when trying for additional conceptions in future years.

IVF has been shown to be effective for patients with PCOS, as they typically have a favorable response with higher numbers of mature oocytes retrieved and increased clinical pregnancy rates. However, individuals with PCOS have an increased risk of ovarian hyperstimulation syndrome (OHSS), and therefore, planning their IVF cycle should assess and address that risk. Selecting a starting gonadotropin dose should consider age and anti-mullerian hormone level. When used in an antagonist protocol, the option for a gonadotropin-releasing hormone–agonist trigger can nearly eliminate the risk of severe OHSS. Those at the highest risk should also consider freezing all embryos and planning a frozen embryo transfer in the following month. Planning for a frozen embryo transfer will not only minimize the risk of OHSS but it may also increase the chances of a successful pregnancy.[35] Additionally, frozen embryo transfer is required in patients who elect for preimplantation genetic testing (PGT). However, neither the diagnosis of PCOS nor obesity has shown higher rates of embryonic aneuploidy. Thus, the decision for PGT is an elective, personal decision in the absence of other conditions, such as single gene mutations, recurrent pregnancy loss, advanced maternal age, and so forth.

SUMMARY

In summary, caring for women with PCOS requires thoughtful attention to the symptoms that are most concerning to the individual, a comprehensive evaluation, and a multidisciplinary approach to treatment. Care should be empathetic and creative so that every woman receives thorough education and an individualized treatment plan.

DISCLOSURE

The authors have nothing to disclose.

REFERENCES

1. Fritz MA, Speroff L. Clinical gynecologic endocrinology and infertility. 8th edition. Philadelphia, PA: Lippincott Williams & Wilkins; 2011. p. 489.
2. Woolcock J, Critchley HO, Munro MG. Review of the confusion in current and historical terminology and definitions for disturbances of menstrual bleeding. Fertil Steril 2008;89(5):1250–9. https://doi.org/10.1016/j.fertnstert.2008.02.096.
3. Costello MF, Shrestha B, Eden J, et al. Metformin versus oral contraceptive pill in polycystic ovary syndrome: a Cochrane review. Hum Reprod 2007;22(5):1200–9.
4. Oguz SH, Yildiz BO. An Update on Contraception in Polycystic Ovary Syndrome. Endocrinol Metab (Seoul) 2021;36(2):296–311.
5. Legro RS, Barnhart HX, Schlaff WD, et al. alClomiphene, metformin, or both for infertility in the polycystic ovary syndrome. N Engl J Med 2007;356(6):551–66.
6. Teede HJ, Misso ML, Costello MF, et al, PCOS Network. Recommendations from the international evidence-based guideline for the assessment and management of polycystic ovary syndrome. Hum Reprod 2018;33(9):1602–18. Erratum in: Hum Reprod. 2019 Feb 1;34(2):388. PMID: 30052961; PMCID: PMC6112576.
7. New MI. Nonclassic 21-hydroxylase deficiency. Fertil Steril 2006 Jul;86(Suppl 1):S2.

8. Pinola P, Piltonen TT, Puurunen J, et al. Androgen Profile Through Life in Women With Polycystic Ovary Syndrome: A Nordic Multicenter Collaboration Study. J Clin Endocrinol Metab 2015;100(9):3400–7.

9. Legro RS, Gnatuk CL, Kunselman AR, et al. Changes in glucose tolerance over time in women with polycystic ovary syndrome: a controlled study. J Clin Endocrinol Metab 2005 Jun;90(6):3236–42.

10. Hudecova M, Holte J, Olovsson M, et al. Diabetes and impaired glucose tolerance in patients with polycystic ovary syndrome–a long term follow-up. Hum Reprod 2011 Jun;26(6):1462–8.

11. Gambineri A, Patton L, Altieri P, et al. Polycystic ovary syndrome is a risk factor for type 2 diabetes: results from a long-term prospective study. Diabetes 2012 Sep; 61(9):2369–74.

12. Schmidt J, Landin-Wilhelmsen K, Brännström M, et al. Cardiovascular disease and risk factors in PCOS women of postmenopausal age: a 21-year controlled follow-up study. J Clin Endocrinol Metab 2011 Dec;96(12):3794–803.

13. Sam S. Adiposity and metabolic dysfunction in polycystic ovary syndrome. Horm Mol Biol Clin Invest 2015 Feb;21(2):107–16.

14. Gourgari E, Lodish M, Shamburek R, et al. Lipoprotein Particles in Adolescents and Young Women With PCOS Provide Insights Into Their Cardiovascular Risk. J Clin Endocrinol Metabol 2015;100(11):4291–8.

15. Lim SS, Hutchison SK, Van Ryswyk E, et al. Lifestyle changes in women with polycystic ovary syndrome. Cochrane Database Syst Rev 2019 Mar 28;3(3): CD007506.

16. Gu Y, Zhou G, Zhou F, et al. Life Modifications and PCOS: Old Story But New Tales. Front Endocrinol 2022;13:808898.

17. Dos Santos IK, Ashe MC, Cobucci RN, et al. The effect of exercise as an intervention for women with polycystic ovary syndrome: A systematic review and meta-analysis. Medicine (Baltim) 2020 Apr;99(16):e19644.

18. Elkind-Hirsch KE, Chappell N, et al. Liraglutide 3 mg on weight, body composition, and hormonal and metabolic parameters in women with obesity and polycystic ovary syndrome: a randomized placebo-controlled-phase 3 study. Fertil Steril 2022 Aug;118(2):371–81.

19. Barry JA, Kuczmierczyk AR, Hardiman PJ. Anxiety and depression in polycystic ovary syndrome: a systematic review and meta-analysis. Hum Reprod 2011 Sep; 26(9):2442–51.

20. Greff D, Juhász AE, Váncsa S, et al. Inositol is an effective and safe treatment in polycystic ovary syndrome: a systematic review and meta-analysis of randomized controlled trials. Reprod Biol Endocrinol 2023 Jan 26;21(1):10.

21. Cooney LG, Lee I, Sammel MD, et al. High prevalence of moderate and severe depressive and anxiety symptoms in polycystic ovary syndrome: a systematic review and meta-analysis. Hum Reprod 2017 May 1;32(5):1075–91.

22. Dokras A, Clifton S, Futterweit W, et al. Increased risk for abnormal depression scores in women with polycystic ovary syndrome: a systematic review and meta-analysis. Obstet Gynecol Surv 2011;66(9):630–8.

23. Himelein MJ, Thatcher SS. Polycystic ovary syndrome and mental health: a review. Obstet Gynecol Surv 2006;61(11):723–32.

24. Teede HJ, Joham AE, Paul E, et al. Longitudinal weight gain in women identified with polycystic ovary syndrome: results of an observational study in young women. Obesity 2013;21(8):1526–32.

25. Trent ME, Rich M, Austin SB, et al. Quality of life in adolescent girls with polycystic ovary syndrome. Arch Pediatr Adolesc Med 2002;156(6):556–60.

26. Ahmed MI, Ahmed M, Saeed M, et al. The efficacy of antidepressants for depression in women with polycystic ovary syndrome: a systematic review and meta-analysis. Endocr Connect 2017;6(8):647–58.
27. Bazarganipour F, Ziaei S, Montazeri A, et al. Psychological investigation in patients with polycystic ovary syndrome. Health Qual Life Outcomes 2013;11:141.
28. McGovern PG, Legro RS, Myers ER, et al. Utility of screening for other causes of infertility in women with "known" polycystic ovary syndrome. Fertil Steril 2007 Feb; 87(2):442–4.
29. Cena H, Chiovato L, Nappi RE. Obesity, Polycystic Ovary Syndrome, and Infertility: A New Avenue for GLP-1 Receptor Agonists. J Clin Endocrinol Metab 2020 Aug 1;105(8):e2695–709.
30. Legro RS, Dodson WC, Kunselman AR, et al. Randomized controlled trial of preconception interventions in infertile women with polycystic ovary syndrome. J Clin Endocrinol Metabol 2015;100(11):4048–58.
31. Legro RS, Brzyski RG, Diamond MP, et al. Letrozole versus clomiphene for infertility in the polycystic ovary syndrome. N Engl J Med 2014;371(2):119–29.
32. Legro RS, Barnhart HX, Schlaff WD, et al. Clomiphene, metformin, or both for infertility in the polycystic ovary syndrome. N Engl J Med 2007;356(6):551–66.
33. Mejia RB, Summers KM, Kresowik JD, et al. A randomized controlled trial of combination letrozole and clomiphene citrate or letrozole alone for ovulation induction in women with polycystic ovary syndrome. Fertil Steril 2019 Mar;111(3):571–8.e1.
34. Peng G, Yan Z, Liu Y, et al. The effects of first-line pharmacological treatments for reproductive outcomes in infertile women with PCOS: a systematic review and network meta-analysis. Reprod Biol Endocrinol 2023;21:24.
35. Chen ZJ, Shi Y, Sun Y, et al. Fresh versus Frozen Embryos for Infertility in the Polycystic Ovary Syndrome. N Engl J Med 2016;375(6):523–33.

Planned Oocyte Cryopreservation

A Review of Current Evidence on Outcomes, Safety and Risks

Bonnie B. Song, MD[a],*, Molly M. Quinn, MD[a,b]

KEYWORDS

- Oocyte cryopreservation • Fertility preservation • Oocyte yield • Vitrification
- Slow freezing • Reproductive outcomes • Elective egg freezing

KEY POINTS

- Oocyte vitrification is an effective method for fertility preservation. An increasing number of oocyte cryopreservation cycles have been documented since the treatment was deemed no longer experimental in 2013. However, few patients have returned to use their cryopreserved oocytes.
- Black and Hispanic patients have lower utilization of planned oocyte cryopreservation compared with White and Asian patients but oocyte yield does not seem to differ significantly by race or ethnicity.
- Live birth rates from the use of cryopreserved oocytes vary with age and number of oocytes frozen, although evidence to predict likelihood of live birth for a given individual is limited.
- Neonatal and obstetric outcomes seem similar after the use of vitrified oocytes compared with in vitro fertilization with fresh oocytes.
- A minority of patients face decision regret after freezing their oocytes but most women report satisfaction with their decision.

INTRODUCTION

Oocyte cryopreservation is a form of assisted reproductive technology that aims to preserve fertility by freezing gametes for future use. Many advances have been made in oocyte cryopreservation since the first birth from a frozen oocyte in 1986. Although initially used as a fertility preservation strategy before receiving gonadotoxic

[a] University of Southern California/Los Angeles General Medical Center, 2051 Marengo Street, Los Angeles, CA 90033, USA; [b] HRC Fertility, 55 S Lake Avenue, Suite 900, Pasadena, CA 91101, USA
* Corresponding author. University of Southern California/Los Angeles General Medical Center, 1200 North State Street, IPT C3F107, Los Angeles, CA 90033.
E-mail address: bonnie.song@med.usc.edu

Obstet Gynecol Clin N Am 50 (2023) 707–719
https://doi.org/10.1016/j.ogc.2023.08.005
0889-8545/23/© 2023 Elsevier Inc. All rights reserved.

treatment in the setting of a cancer diagnosis, oocyte cryopreservation has become increasingly popular among healthy women seeking to preserve their reproductive potential. Fertility decline with advancing maternal age is a relationship that has been well studied.[1] Meanwhile, US societal trends demonstrate an increased rate of delayed childbearing.[2] Thus, it is unsurprising that the number of patients electively pursuing oocyte cryopreservation for social reasons, formally known as planned oocyte cryopreservation (POC), continues to grow.[3] As POC increases in popularity, obstetricians and gynecologists (ob-gyns) should be prepared to discuss fertility preservation options with their patients. However, a recent survey by Fritz and colleagues showed that although ob-gyns agreed that discussions about reproductive aging are important for all reproductive age patients, a majority of respondents reported lacking time or knowledge to counsel their patients about fertility preservation.[4] Because the use of POC is relatively new, initial data describing outcomes and utilization trends are only beginning to emerge. Here we review some of the latest advances and practices in POC as well as preliminary evidence on reproductive outcomes. We will also review data on the safety, benefits, and risks of POC. The aim of this narrative review is to inform providers of recent advances in POC and synthesize recent literature important for counseling patients considering oocyte cryopreservation to defer childbearing.

OOCYTE CRYOPRESERVATION: A BRIEF HISTORY

The first publication of a successful pregnancy from a frozen–thawed oocyte was made in 1986.[5] This was followed by rare reports of successful pregnancies following in vitro fertilization (IVF) of vitrified oocytes in subsequent years of continuous efforts. Slow freezing techniques, which allow for cryopreservation to occur at a sufficiently slow rate to permit cellular dehydration while minimizing intracellular ice formation, was the predominant method used for many years with limited success.[6] This trend began to change with the introduction of vitrification, with the first neonate born following the use of this technology in 1999.

Vitrification involves an instant rapid freezing from liquid to glass state without allowing the formation of ice crystals that could destroy the delicate oocyte.[7] To minimize cryodamage during this process, various substances are used, which typically include a mix of permeable and nonpermeable cryoprotectants. However, cryoprotectants can also cause cellular damage including direct toxicity and osmotic injury.[8,9] To ameliorate individual cryoprotectant toxicity, multiple cryoprotectants can be used at lower concentrations.[10] With the emergence of more refined vitrification protocols in the past decade, vitrification success rates have markedly improved and vitrification is currently the cryopreservation technique of choice today.[8,11–13] Overall, survival rates of oocytes thawed after vitrification range from 80% to 90%, although this can vary with age.[14] Thawed oocytes are subsequently fertilized using intracytoplasmic sperm injection (ICSI) to overcome hardening of the zona pellucida following cryopreservation, with fertilization rates varying between 70% and 80%.[14] Although vitrification is currently a fully hands-on procedure, attempts to at least partially automate the process are underway.[15–17] Benefits of vitrification are further demonstrated when cryopreserving biopsied embryos. With slow freezing, many biopsied embryos do not survive a subsequent thaw. Among those that do, many of the cells degenerate, resulting in a decrease in embryo viability.[8,18] However, when vitrified biopsied embryos are warmed, embryos survive virtually intact.[18]

Coincident with the transition from slow freeze to vitrification, in 2013, the American Society for Reproductive Medicine (ASRM) designated oocyte cryopreservation no longer experimental based on its use for fertility preservation in oncology patients.[19]

In 2018, the ASRM practice committee described social egg freezing as ethically permissible, terming it "planned oocyte cryopreservation."[20] During the past decade, utilization of oocyte cryopreservation has grown exponentially. In the United States, fertility preservation cycles increased from 2227 in 2013 to 16,194 in 2019.[3,21]

CURRENT EVIDENCE ON PLANNED OOCYTE CRYOPRESERVATION
Fertility Preservation Treatment Outcomes

Oocyte yield
Consistent with data from autologous IVF for any indication, the primary predictor of oocyte yield following ovarian stimulation for fertility preservation is age at oocyte retrieval. Doyle and colleagues did not find any significant differences in oocyte yield, implantation, or birth outcome between patients pursing oocyte vitrification electively or for infertility.[22] However, authors did note that patients pursuing elective fertility preservation were significantly older at the times of oocyte vitrification (by 4.3 years) and warming (by 5.7 years). Another study by Cobo and colleagues comparing patients pursuing fertility preservation electively versus before cancer treatment found that oocyte yield was higher per cycle among patients with cancer (9.6 vs 11.4) but the difference was no longer significant after correcting for age of participants.[23] Kasaven and colleagues found that among 373 women pursuing POC, each increase in age of 1 year resulted in a 4% reduction in oocyte yield after adjusting for all other variables. The authors also found that body mass index (BMI), estradiol levels on the day of trigger, and the number of follicles greater than 12 mm at trigger were all significant predictors of yield at retrieval.[24] Although this study showed an associated increase in oocyte yield with an increased BMI within a cohort of women of majority normal BMI (20–24.9), other studies of patients undergoing IVF for any indication have shown that oocyte quantity is not significantly affected by BMI, suggesting that further studies are needed to better understand the influence of BMI on oocyte yield and reproductive outcomes for patients undergoing POC.[25,26]

Utilization rates
A retrospective cohort analysis by Katler and colleagues of oocyte preservation cycles between 2012 and 2016 showed that the majority of oocyte cryopreservation cycles were performed in White patients (66.5%), although the number of oocyte cryopreservation cycles increased annually among all ethnic groups, with the fastest growth among Asian patients.[27] Furthermore, the age of oocyte cryopreservation among patients of all ethnic backgrounds was on average less than 35 years, and patients underwent an average of 1.28 oocyte cryopreservation cycles. Asian patients most commonly underwent oocyte cryopreservation at an average age between 35 and 37 years and were more likely to have undergone 2 or more cycles than patients of other minority groups. After adjustment for cofounders, authors found no clinically significant differences in oocyte yield and percentage of maturation across racial and ethnic groups. However, when stratifying the proportion of oocyte preservation cycles by minority status compared with the background demographics of the US population, oocyte cryopreservation was underutilized by Black and Hispanic patients. Similarly, Yilmaz and colleagues found that Black and Hispanic patients underwent POC at lower rates, making up 3.8% and 2.5%, respectively, of the Society for Assisted Reproductive Technology Clinic Outcome and Reporting System Database, compared with White (36%) and Asian (10.4%) patients.[28] There are likely numerous potential explanations for these differences in utilization of oocyte cryopreservation but differences in access to fertility care, such as insurance coverage, proximity to fertility clinics, and sociodemographic stratification, are important factors to consider.

Outcomes following POC are emerging as patients within the past decade return to use their frozen oocytes. **Table 1** provides an overview comparing outcomes among 8 cohort analyses collecting similar data including mean age of patients at their first retrieval for POC, mean number of vitrified oocytes, mean number of cycles per patient, percentage of patients returning to use their oocytes, percentage of patients with a live birth. Current studies show that most women who underwent POC have not returned to thaw their oocytes, with return rates varying from 4.6% to 38%.[24,29–37] Notably, women who underwent POC seem to still have significantly higher utilization rates than patients with cancer pursuing fertility preservation according to a study by Cobo and colleagues (12.1 vs 7.4%).[23] The most commonly reported reason for not using stored oocytes was not wanting to be a single parent, followed by desire to try to conceive naturally, and not wanting to use a sperm donor.[38] Return rates of patients presenting to thaw their oocytes seem similar by age group at freezing.[29] Notably, a retrospective study of oocyte thaw outcomes found that the number of oocytes thawed to achieve pregnancy and live birth increased significantly with increasing age at the time of cryopreservation.[39] Furthermore, among pregnancies resulting from thawed oocytes, the rate of good perinatal outcomes decreased as the age at time of cryopreservation increased.[39]

Reproductive outcomes and fertility preservation outcome prediction models

A recent prospective study surveying 228 women who underwent POC found that 101 (44%) tried to conceive during the study period of 2009 to 2015 and 66 (65%) became pregnant. Within the group of women who became pregnant, most (76%) conceived naturally, whereas 7% conceived through ICSI injection with their vitrified oocytes, and 17% by other medically assisted reproduction treatments.[40] The median time to follow-up of these patients was 31 months.

Age at time of egg freezing and the number of stored oocytes are key factors that affect later reproductive outcomes. Knowledge of these predictors has led to recommendations on optimal timelines for POC.[22,41] Per the ESHRE Guideline Group on Fertility Preservation, the optimal age for a woman to freeze her eggs with significantly higher success rates is younger than 35 years, before the quality and number of eggs decline.[42] Multiple studies estimate that on average, freezing 20 oocytes is optimal to achieve pregnancy; whereas a minimum of 8 to 10 oocytes are recommended.[22,23,43,44] Maslow and colleaguesfound that of 1241 patients undergoing POC, for those who underwent 1 egg freezing cycle, 66% achieved a 50% or greater estimated live birth rate and 51% achieved 70% or greater estimated live birth rate.[45] With 2 cycles, 79.6% of patients attained a 50% or greater estimated live birth rate and 65% achieved a 70% or greater estimated live birth rate. Authors reported that achieving a 50%, 60%, or 70% estimated live birth rate within 1 to 2 cycles was significantly associated with age and anti-Mullerian hormone (AMH) levels.[45] Age younger than 37.5 years and AMH greater than 1.995 were independently associated with attaining 60% estimated live birth rate with 1 cycle. Per analyses by Cobo and colleagues success rates for a live birth reach a plateau past a certain number of oocytes frozen.[23] This plateau was reached among women aged 35 years and younger at 24 oocytes, with a cumulative probability of live birth of 94.4%. Conversely, at 8 to 10 oocytes, the cumulative probability was 32% to 42.8% in this age group. Among women older than 35 years, live birth rate plateaued at 20 oocytes (cumulative probability 49.5%) while the probability of live birth at 8 to 10 used oocytes was 17.3% to 25.2%. Based on extrapolation of available outcomes data from oocyte cryopreservation cycles and autologous IVF cycles for any indication, models have been developed to help predict how many oocytes, and therefore, cycles might be needed for patients

Table 1
Cohort analyses of reproductive outcomes

Study	Study Type	Setting	POC Population Size	Study Period	Patients Returning to Use Oocytes (%)	Patients with Live Births (%)[c]	Mean Age at First Retrieval	Mean Number of Vitrified Oocytes per Cycle	Mean Number of Cycles
Blakemore et al,[29] 2021	Retrospective cohort	Single US large urban university affiliated fertility center	231	10–15 y follow-up of patients pursuing POC 2005–2009	88 (38%)	27 (33.8%)	38.2	11.6	1.2
Cobo et al,[23] 2018	Retrospective cohort	Multicenter, Instituto Valenciano de Infertilidad clinics in Spain	5289	January 2007–May 2018	641 (12.1%)	115[b] total live births	37.2	7.3	1.4
Garcia-Velasco et al,[31] 2013	Retrospective cohort	Multiple university affiliated infertility clinics	560	March 2007–June 2012	26 (4.6%)	5 (19.2%)	36.7	8.1	1.2
Kasaven et al,[24] 2022	Retrospective cohort	Single clinic in London	373	2008–2018	36 (9.7%)	11 (30.5%)	38.3[a]	8[a]	1.14[a]
Leung et al,[33] 2021	Retrospective cohort	Single large university affiliated fertility clinic	921	June 2006–October 2020	68 (7.8)	22 (32.4%)	36.6	12.2	1.4
Nagy et al,[36] 2017	Prospective cohort	16 US infertility clinics	46	June 2008–September 2010	—	8 (17.4%)	33.9	9.2	1.0
Wennberg et al,[32] 2019	Retrospective cohort	Nordic IVF Göteborg	254	August 2011–August 2017	38 (15.0%)	5 total[b] live births	36.9	5.4	1.4
Yang et al,[35] 2022	Retrospective cohort	Single medical center in Taipei, Taiwan	645	November 2002–December 2020	54 (8.4%)	17 (31.5%)	37.5	11	1.3

[a] Only medians were reported.
[b] Only total live births were reported number of patients with live births unknown.
[c] Patients with live births from using banked oocytes.

to achieve their fertility goals.[22,46] Doyle and colleagues reviewed all oocyte retrievals for autologous IVF conducted from 2009 to 2013 to derive age-related probabilities of having at least 1, 2, or 3 live born children according to the number of oocytes cryopreserved.[36] Goldman and colleagues extrapolated data from ICSI cycles in infertility patients to help predict the number of cycles that would be needed and the probability of a woman having at least 1, 2, or 3 live births.[46] Such models can aid as counseling tools to help provide reasonable expectations regarding the number of mature cryopreserved oocytes potentially needed for patients to reach their family building goals. Notably, although these models can be helpful counseling tools, they were developed based off of retrospective data, sometimes from a single institution. The data used and assumptions made to create these models may not directly applicable to different patient populations.

Indications for Planned Oocyte Cryopreservation

Studies report that the most common indication for elective oocyte preservation is not having a partner.[47,48] In a retrospective observational study by Cobo and colleagues, of 79% of women who were single at the time of cryopreservation, 47% were partnered by the time they returned to use their eggs, suggesting the potential significance of elective oocyte preservation among single women.[41] Similarly, in a recent retrospective study by Gurtin and colleagues, among patients who froze their eggs for "social" reasons, 97.8% were single at the time of first freeze and 52% of this group was in a heterosexual relationship when they came back to thaw their eggs.[49] The second most commonly observed reason for POC is professional, with patients reporting desire for education completion, for career advancement, or inflexibility in the workplace.[50–52] A recent study of the psychosocial determinants influencing Australian women's intentions to freeze their eggs showed that the strongest behavioral belief of participants was "reducing anxiety and regrets about my future so I don't 'miss out.'"[53]

Risks and Safety

Fertility preservation counseling should involve shared decision-making that considers the risks and benefits associated with POC. Risks include those inherent to ovarian stimulation and oocyte retrieval. The most common risk is that of ovarian hyperstimulation syndrome (OHSS), which is reduced in POC because there is no embryo transfer at the end of the stimulation cycle. Gonadotropin releasing hormone agonist triggers, used in the context of gonadotropin releasing hormone antagonist cycles, can further decrease the chance of development of ovarian hyperstimulation.[54] Kasaven and colleagues reported 4%, or 9 of 373 cases of OHSS among women undergoing POC, all defined as mild severity per the Royal college of Obstetrician and Gynecologist classification.[24] Oocyte retrieval procedures might result in intraperitoneal bleeding, pelvic infection, damage to surrounding organs, ovarian torsion, and anesthesia risks, all of which are uncommon. These risks are reported to affect 0.76% of patients undergoing oocyte stimulation and retrieval, with hospital admission necessary for 0.56% of patients.[55] The risk of bleeding is higher after more than 30 oocytes are retrieved.[56]

Because vitrification was adopted only within the last dozen years, there are scarce data on long-term safety with respect to offspring health. More time is needed for significant numbers of women to return to use their cryopreserved oocytes and for their frozen oocyte-derived offspring to age. A recent retrospective study using Danish registry data found that use of frozen *embryo* transfer was associated with a small but statistically significant elevated risk of childhood cancer, particularly with leukemia and neuroblastoma compared with naturally conceived children.[57] The absolute risk remained extremely low, and findings have been questioned for various reasons, including study design, differences in group sizes, and low prevalence of disease finding. Furthermore, a majority of the included cases was based on slow freezing, and data may not be pertinent to vitrification.[57] Some studies report that frozen embryo transfer is associated with large for gestational age and higher mean birth weight compared to fresh embryo transfer, suggesting that techniques involving cryopreservation may induce changes in the developing embryo that affect intrauterine growth.[58,59] However, there are also reports showing no difference between fresh and frozen embryo transfer regarding the birth weight of infants from IVF cycles.[60,61] Furthermore, these data are investigating the influence of embryo freezing techniques on subsequent live birth and childhood outcomes and not a frozen oocyte, which is subsequently fertilized and may be transferred fresh.

Another risk to consider is the maternal risks of an advanced maternal age pregnancy. A recent UK study of 85 women who underwent elective egg freezing between 2008 and 2018 found that 72% of participants were aware of the elevated risks of preeclampsia, pulmonary embolism, and preterm birth with advanced maternal age; however, 83% of participants accepted these risks in order to become pregnant at a more suitable time.[62] Furthermore, POC may give women and couples a sense of false security, and women may rely too confidently on their preserved oocytes. Studies have consistently showed that patients overestimate success rates of assisted reproductive technology.[47,53,63] A recent cohort study showed the success rate of POC was overestimated in 72% of participants.[47] Similarly, Greenwood and colleagues found that a recent survey of respondents between the ages of 34 and 40 years estimated an average 56% probability of achieving live birth with their cryopreserved oocytes,[63] an overestimation given available outcomes data.[29,64] Furthermore, 13 of the women surveyed (6%) estimated a 100% likelihood of having a baby with their banked oocytes, which presents a critical opportunity for counseling. Further age-stratified investigations are needed to describe the number of oocytes required to produce acceptable likelihoods for pregnancy and live birth.[46,65,66]

Decision regret is a risk that could result from the rapid uptake of POC. A recent study surveying patients who underwent POC found that 49% of women had some degree of decision regret, whereas 16% had moderate-to-severe regret.[63] Those in the lowest quartile of total eggs banked (10 or less) had a 4-fold increased odds of regret compared with those freezing more than 10 oocytes. Women who perceived lower adequacy of information and emotional support during the treatment process were also significantly more likely to experience regret. Although the majority reported that they had adequate information before the process and 69% perceived adequate emotional support, 20% of respondents did not report that they received adequate counseling or emotional support, suggesting an opportunity for improvement in patient care.[63]

Outside of considerations for the risk of decision regret, risks inherent to ovarian stimulation and oocyte retrieval, and risks of an advanced maternal age (AMA) pregnancy, the risks inherent to POC are low. No known risks specific to freezing have been noted, and the time in storage does not seem to affect reproductive outcomes.[67–69] Additionally, using vitrified oocytes do not seem to negatively influence neonatal outcomes. Birth reports indicate no increase in aneuploidy rates or congenital abnormalities in infants from cryopreserved oocytes compared with IVF-conceived infants, and there is no association with further obstetric or perinatal morbidity.[68,70–72] Two recent studies following children born from vitrified-warmed oocytes have been promising. Van Reckem and colleagues found that the health outcomes of 72 two-year-old children born after oocyte vitrification were similar compared with those born after fresh IVF with embryo transfer.[73] Takeshige and colleagues also found that the mental and physical development of 282 children born after oocyte vitrification was comparable to that of children conceived naturally in a 6-year follow-up study.[74] From a cost–benefit perspective, depending on age, POC could be of greater value compared with conventional IVF.[65,75] For women desiring to defer pregnancy until the age of 40 years, oocyte cryopreservation before the age of 38 years reduces the overall cost to obtain a live birth.[65]

DISCUSSION

Setting patient expectations based on current reproductive outcomes and counseling patients about the risks, safety, and benefits of POC is important. The ASRM Ethics Committee stated that POC is compatible with the principles of beneficence because the intervention could potentially be a primary preventative strategy for age-related fertility decline.[20,64] Similar to contraceptive choice, oocyte cryopreservation can also enhance reproductive autonomy, allowing women more time to have and raise children at a time they perceive optimal. POC reduces the pressure to have a child when women are not yet psychologically, socially, or situationally ready. In a recent study by Seyhan and colleagues, 98.8% of women surveyed who cryopreserved oocytes for nonmedical indications reported they would recommend oocyte cryopreservation to a friend, and 72% reported they felt more secure in terms of their reproductive potential.[47] Additionally, 89% of women surveyed reported satisfaction with their decision to freeze their eggs, even if they never use them.[63] Patients should be relayed such information regarding satisfaction and safety of POC while also considering the lack of data on long-term outcomes of children born from vitrified oocytes. Furthermore, after informing patients on the risks of decision regret, providers should also ensure patients have adequate emotional support and counseling on their likelihood of having a live birth. They should provide recommendations on the number of oocytes to freeze and potential need for undergoing multiple cycles based on their family-building goals. Ultimately, shared decision-making to assess the value POC may or may not have for a particular patient will be of primary importance in counseling.

SUMMARY

The development and refinement of vitrification techniques during the past 15 years have markedly improved the success of oocyte cryopreservation. Oocyte cryopreservation was initially used for fertility preservation before undergoing gonadotoxic treatments but is now becoming increasingly used to circumvent age-related infertility. Because POC is relatively new and most patients who undergo POC have not yet returned to use their oocytes, large-scale outcomes data are relatively sparse. Higher oocyte yield and higher subsequent live birth rates are observed among those who pursue POC at younger ages, reenforcing the effect of age on fertility preservation outcomes. Meanwhile, race and ethnicity do not seem to affect oocyte yield, although POC is underutilized among Black and Hispanic patients. Patients may overestimate the success of their cryopreserved oocytes, suggesting a need for individualizable counseling tools to help patients predict the number of cryopreserved oocytes needed for an acceptable likelihood of a live birth. Although there is limited evidence to predict the likelihood of live birth in women undergoing POC, preliminary models offering guidance on the optimal number of oocytes to cryopreserve to reach fertility goals have been proposed.[22,46] As we continue to build data on reproductive outcomes over time and better understand the effect of factors such as BMI, smoking or ethnicity, we can also provide more concrete guidance to patients. Furthermore, as rates of delayed childbearing continue to increase, it is more important than ever for providers to incorporate counseling about POC into routine discussions with patients about their reproductive life plans.

CLINICS CARE POINTS

- Most women who underwent POC have not returned to thaw their oocytes, with return rates varying from 4.6% to 38%.

- The optimal age for a woman to freeze her eggs with significantly higher success rates is less than 35 years, before the quality and number of eggs decline.

- On average, freezing 20 oocytes is optimal to achieve pregnancy, whereas a minimum of 8 to 10 oocytes are recommended, although these numbers do vary with age.

- Long-term data on risks of POC on offspring health are scarce but no known risks specific to freezing have been noted and vitrified oocytes do not seem to negatively affect neonatal outcomes.

- Moderate-to-severe decision regret has been noted in a minority of participants, with those freezing 10 or less oocytes and those who perceived lower adequacy of information and emotional support being more likely to experience regret.

DISCLOSURE

The authors declare that they have no relevant or material financial interests that relate to the research described in this article.

REFERENCES

1. Schwartz D, Mayaux MJ. Female fecundity as a function of age: results of artificial insemination in 2193 nulliparous women with azoospermic husbands. Federation CECOS. N Engl J Med. 1982;306(7):404–6.
2. Products - Data Briefs - Number 232 - January 2016. Published June 8, 2019. Available at: https://www.cdc.gov/nchs/products/databriefs/db232.htm. Accessed November 7, 2022.
3. More Than 73 Thousand Babies Born from Assisted Reproductive Technology Cycles Done in 2020. Available at: https://www.asrm.org/news-and-publications/news-and-research/press-releases-and-bulletins/more-than-73-thousand-babies-born-from-assisted-reproductive-technology-cycles-done-in-2020/. Accessed October 10, 2022.
4. Fritz R, Klugman S, Lieman H, et al. Counseling patients on reproductive aging and elective fertility preservation-a survey of obstetricians and gynecologists' experience, approach, and knowledge. J Assist Reprod Genet 2018;35(9): 1613–21.
5. Chen C. PREGNANCY AFTER HUMAN OOCYTE CRYOPRESERVATION. Lancet 1986;327(8486):884–6.
6. Bernard A, Fuller B. Cryopreservation of human oocytes: a review of current problems and perspectives. Hum Reprod Update 1996;2(3):193–207.
7. Fahy GM, Wowk B. Principles of Ice-Free Cryopreservation by Vitrification. Methods Mol Biol 2021;2180:27–97.
8. Nagy ZP, Shapiro D, Chang CC. Vitrification of the human embryo: a more efficient and safer in vitro fertilization treatment. Fertil Steril 2020;113(2):241–7.

9. El Cury-Silva T, Nunes MEG, Casalechi M, et al. Cryoprotectant agents for ovarian tissue vitrification: Systematic review. Cryobiology 2021;103:7–14.

10. Chang CC, Shapiro DB, Nagy ZP. The effects of vitrification on oocyte quality. Biol Reprod 2022;106(2):316–27.

11. Cobo A, García-Velasco JA, Remohí J, et al. Oocyte vitrification for fertility preservation for both medical and nonmedical reasons. Fertil Steril 2021;115(5): 1091–101.

12. Rienzi L, Gracia C, Maggiulli R, et al. Oocyte, embryo and blastocyst cryopreservation in ART: systematic review and meta-analysis comparing slow-freezing versus vitrification to produce evidence for the development of global guidance. Hum Reprod Update 2017;23(2):139–55.

13. Hanson BM, Kim JG, Suarez SI, et al. Embryology outcomes after oocyte vitrification with super-cooled slush nitrogen are similar to outcomes with conventional liquid nitrogen: a randomized controlled trial. Fertil Steril 2022;117(1):106–14.

14. Saumet J, Petropanagos A, Buzaglo K, et al. No. 356-Egg Freezing for Age-Related Fertility Decline. J Obstet Gynaecol Can 2018;40(3):356–68.

15. Gatimel N, Moreau J, Bettiol C, et al. Semi-automated versus manual embryo vitrification: inter-operator variability, time-saving, and clinical outcomes. J Assist Reprod Genet 2021;38(12):3213–22.

16. Koning RI, Vader H, van Nugteren M, et al. Automated vitrification of cryo-EM samples with controllable sample thickness using suction and real-time optical inspection. Nat Commun 2022;13(1):2985.

17. Miao S, Jiang Z, Luo J, et al. A Robotic System with Embedded Open Microfluidic Chip for Automatic Embryo Vitrification. IEEE Trans Biomed Eng 2022. https://doi. org/10.1109/TBME.2022.3171628. PP.

18. Keskintepe L, Sher G, Machnicka A, et al. Vitrification of human embryos subjected to blastomere biopsy for pre-implantation genetic screening produces higher survival and pregnancy rates than slow freezing. J Assist Reprod Genet 2009;26(11–12):629–35.

19. Practice Committees of the American Society for Reproductive Medicine and the Society for Assisted Reproductive Technology. Mature oocyte cryopreservation: a guideline. Fertil Steril 2013;99(1):37–43.

20. Daar J, Benward J, Collins L, et al. Planned oocyte cryopreservation for women seeking to preserve future reproductive potential: an Ethics Committee opinion. Fertil Steril 2018;110(6):1022–8.

21. National Summary Report Available at: https://www.sartcorsonline.com/Csr/ Public?ClinicPKID=0#patient-cumulative. Accessed January 7, 2023.

22. Doyle JO, Richter KS, Lim J, et al. Successful elective and medically indicated oocyte vitrification and warming for autologous in vitro fertilization, with predicted birth probabilities for fertility preservation according to number of cryopreserved oocytes and age at retrieval. Fertil Steril 2016;105(2):459–66.e2.

23. Cobo A, García-Velasco J, Domingo J, et al. Elective and Onco-fertility preservation: factors related to IVF outcomes. Hum Reprod 2018;33(12):2222–31.

24. Kasaven LS, Jones BP, Heath C, et al. Reproductive outcomes from ten years of elective oocyte cryopreservation. Arch Gynecol Obstet 2022;306(5):1753–60.

25. Banker M, Sorathiya D, Shah S. Effect of Body Mass Index on the Outcome of In-Vitro Fertilization/Intracytoplasmic Sperm Injection in Women. J Hum Reprod Sci 2017;10(1):37–43.

26. Christensen MW, Ingerslev HJ, Degn B, et al. Effect of Female Body Mass Index on Oocyte Quantity in Fertility Treatments (IVF): Treatment Cycle Number Is a

Possible Effect Modifier. A Register-Based Cohort Study. PLoS One 2016;11(9): e0163393.

27. Katler QS, Shandley LM, Hipp HS, et al. National egg-freezing trends: cycle and patient characteristics with a focus on race/ethnicity. Fertil Steril 2021;116(2): 528–37.

28. Yilmaz BD, Muhammad LN, Yeh C, et al. Does racial disparity exist in planned oocyte cryopreservation cycles? a sart database analysis of 15,806 CYCLES. Fertil Steril 2022;118(4 Supplement):e84.

29. Blakemore JK, Grifo JA, DeVore SM, et al. Planned oocyte cryopreservation—10–15-year follow-up: return rates and cycle outcomes. Fertil Steril 2021;115(6): 1511–20.

30. Cobo A, Garcia-Velasco JA, Domingo J, et al. Is vitrification of oocytes useful for fertility preservation for age-related fertility decline and in cancer patients? Fertil Steril 2013;99(6):1485–95.

31. Garcia-Velasco JA, Domingo J, Cobo A, et al. Five years' experience using oocyte vitrification to preserve fertility for medical and nonmedical indications. Fertil Steril 2013;99(7):1994–9.

32. Wennberg AL, Schildauer K, Brännström M. Elective oocyte freezing for nonmedical reasons: a 6-year report on utilization and in vitro fertilization results from a Swedish center. Acta Obstet Gynecol Scand 2019;98(11):1429–34.

33. Leung AQ, Baker K, Vaughan D, et al. Clinical outcomes and utilization from over a decade of planned oocyte cryopreservation. Reprod Biomed Online 2021; 43(4):671–9.

34. Schattman GL. Cryopreservation of Oocytes. N Engl J Med 2015;373(18): 1755–60.

35. Yang IJ, Wu MY, Chao KH, et al. Usage and cost-effectiveness of elective oocyte freezing: a retrospective observational study. Reprod Biol Endocrinol 2022; 20:123.

36. Nagy ZP, Anderson RE, Feinberg EC, et al. The Human Oocyte Preservation Experience (HOPE) Registry: evaluation of cryopreservation techniques and oocyte source on outcomes. Reprod Biol Endocrinol 2017;15(1):10.

37. Evidence-based outcomes after oocyte cryopreservation for donor oocyte in vitro fertilization and planned oocyte cryopreservation: a guideline. Fertil Steril 2021; 116(1):36–47.

38. Hammarberg K, Kirkman M, Pritchard N, et al. Reproductive experiences of women who cryopreserved oocytes for non-medical reasons. Hum Reprod 2017;32(3):575–81.

39. Kawwass JF, Crawford S, Hipp HS. Frozen eggs: national autologous oocyte thaw outcomes. Fertil Steril 2021;116(4):1077–84.

40. Balkenende EM, Dahhan T, van der Veen F, et al. Reproductive outcomes after oocyte banking for fertility preservation. Reprod Biomed Online 2018;37(4): 425–33.

41. Cobo A, García-Velasco JA, Coello A, et al. Oocyte vitrification as an efficient option for elective fertility preservation. Fertil Steril 2016;105(3):755–64.e8.

42. Anderson RA, Amant F, Braat D, et al. ESHRE guideline: female fertility preservation. Hum Reprod Open 2020;2020(4):hoaa052.

43. Chronopoulou E, Raperport C, Sfakianakis A, et al. Elective oocyte cryopreservation for age-related fertility decline. J Assist Reprod Genet 2021;38(5):1177–86.

44. Wennberg AL. Social freezing of oocytes: a means to take control of your fertility. Ups J Med Sci 2020;125(2):95–8.

45. Maslow BSL, Guarnaccia MM, Ramirez L, et al. Likelihood of achieving a 50%, 60%, or 70% estimated live birth rate threshold with 1 or 2 cycles of planned oocyte cryopreservation. J Assist Reprod Genet 2020;37(7):1637–43.

46. Goldman RH, Racowsky C, Farland LV, et al. Predicting the likelihood of live birth for elective oocyte cryopreservation: a counseling tool for physicians and patients. Hum Reprod 2017;32(4):853–9.

47. Seyhan A, Akin OD, Ertaş S, et al. A Survey of Women Who Cryopreserved Oocytes for Non-medical Indications (Social Fertility Preservation). Reprod Sci 2021; 28(8):2216–22.

48. Platts S, Trigg B, Bracewell-Milnes T, et al. Exploring women's attitudes, knowledge, and intentions to use oocyte freezing for non-medical reasons: A systematic review. Acta Obstet Gynecol Scand 2021;100(3):383–93.

49. Gürtin ZB, Morgan L, O'Rourke D, et al. For whom the egg thaws: insights from an analysis of 10 years of frozen egg thaw data from two UK clinics, 2008–2017. J Assist Reprod Genet 2019;36(6):1069–80.

50. Alteri A, Pisaturo V, Nogueira D, et al. Elective egg freezing without medical indications. Acta Obstet Gynecol Scand 2019;98(5):647–52.

51. Anderson RA, Davies MC, Lavery SA, et al. Elective Egg Freezing for Non-Medical Reasons: Scientific Impact Paper No. 63. BJOG 2020;127(9):e113–21.

52. Nasab S, Ulin L, Nkele C, et al. Elective egg freezing: what is the vision of women around the globe? Future Sci OA 2020;6(5):FSO468.

53. Caughey LE, White KM. Psychosocial determinants of women's intentions and willingness to freeze their eggs. Fertil Steril 2021;115(3):742–52.

54. Prevention and treatment of moderate and severe ovarian hyperstimulation syndrome: a guideline. Fertil Steril 2016;106(7):1634–47.

55. Levi-Setti PE, Cirillo F, Scolaro V, et al. Appraisal of clinical complications after 23,827 oocyte retrievals in a large assisted reproductive technology program. Fertil Steril 2018;109(6):1038–43.e1.

56. Mizrachi Y, Horowitz E, Farhi J, et al. Ovarian stimulation for freeze-all IVF cycles: a systematic review. Hum Reprod Update 2020;26(1):118–35.

57. Hargreave M, Jensen A, Hansen MK, et al. Association Between Fertility Treatment and Cancer Risk in Children. JAMA 2019;322(22):2203–10.

58. Zhang B, Wei D, Legro RS, et al. Obstetric complications after frozen versus fresh embryo transfer in women with polycystic ovary syndrome: results from a randomized trial. Fertil Steril 2018;109(2):324–9.

59. Terho AM, Pelkonen S, Opdahl S, et al. High birth weight and large-for-gestational-age in singletons born after frozen compared to fresh embryo transfer, by gestational week: a Nordic register study from the CoNARTaS group. Hum Reprod 2021;36(4):1083–92.

60. Besharati M, von Versen-Höynck F, Kapphahn K, et al. Examination of fetal growth trajectories following infertility treatment. J Assist Reprod Genet 2020;37(6): 1399–407.

61. Ainsworth AJ, Wyatt MA, Shenoy CC, et al. Fresh versus frozen embryo transfer has no effect on childhood weight. Fertil Steril 2019;112(4):684–90.e1.

62. Benjamin PJ, Lorraine K, Ariadne L, et al. Perceptions, outcomes, and regret following social egg freezing in the UK; a cross-sectional survey. Acta Obstet Gynecol Scand 2020;99(3).

63. Greenwood EA, Pasch LA, Hastie J, et al. To freeze or not to freeze: decision regret and satisfaction following elective oocyte cryopreservation. Fertil Steril 2018;109(6):1097–104.e1.

64. Goldman KN. Elective oocyte cryopreservation: an ounce of prevention? Fertil Steril 2018;109(6):1014–5.
65. Devine K, Mumford SL, Goldman KN, et al. Baby budgeting: oocyte cryopreservation in women delaying reproduction can reduce cost per live birth. Fertil Steril 2015;103(6):1446–53, e1-2.
66. Mesen TB, Mersereau JE, Kane JB, et al. Optimal timing for elective egg freezing. Fertil Steril 2015;103(6):1551–6.e4.
67. Li J, Yin M, Wang B, et al. The effect of storage time after vitrification on pregnancy and neonatal outcomes among 24 698 patients following the first embryo transfer cycles. Hum Reprod 2020;35(7):1675–84.
68. Gunnala V, Schattman G. Oocyte vitrification for elective fertility preservation: the past, present, and future. Curr Opin Obstet Gynecol 2017;29(1):59–63.
69. Stigliani S, Moretti S, Anserini P, et al. Storage time does not modify the gene expression profile of cryopreserved human metaphase II oocytes. Hum Reprod 2015;30(11):2519–26.
70. Levi-Setti PEP, Borini A, Patrizio P, et al. ART results with frozen oocytes: data from the Italian ART registry (2005–2013). J Assist Reprod Genet 2016;33(1):123–8.
71. Noyes N, Porcu E, Borini A. Over 900 oocyte cryopreservation babies born with no apparent increase in congenital anomalies. Reprod Biomed Online 2009; 18(6):769–76.
72. Tur-Kaspa I, Gal M, Horwitz A. Genetics and health of children born from cryopreserved oocytes. Fertil Steril 2007;88:S14.
73. Van Reckem M, Blockeel C, Bonduelle M, et al. Health of 2-year-old children born after vitrified oocyte donation in comparison with peers born after fresh oocyte donation. Hum Reprod Open 2021;2021(1):hoab002.
74. Takeshige Y, Takahashi M, Hashimoto T, et al. Six-year follow-up of children born from vitrified oocytes. Reprod Biomed Online 2021;42(3):564–71.
75. Fritz R, Jindal S. Reproductive aging and elective fertility preservation. J Ovarian Res 2018;11:66.

Economics of Fertility Care

Benjamin J. Peipert, MD[a], Sloane Mebane, MD[b],
Maxwell Edmonds, MD, PhD[b], Lester Watch, MD[b], Tarun Jain, MD[c],*

KEYWORDS

- Infertility • Access to care • Disparities • Health economics • Health insurance • IVF

KEY POINTS

- In vitro fertilization (IVF) is the most effective infertility treatment; however, medications, diagnostic testing, and procedural costs have made IVF unaffordable for most Americans.
- Preimplantation testing for aneuploidy and intracytoplasmic sperm injection may be cost effective for limited populations, but widespread application of these technologies in clinical practice may be contributing to excessive costs without improvements in patient outcomes.
- State fertility insurance mandates are associated with increased IVF utilization, single embryo transfer rates, decreased multiple gestation rates, and higher live birth rates.
- Expansion of infertility treatment may be a means to combat the declining birth rates while maintaining equitable gender representation in the workforce.

INTRODUCTION

The United States has the most expensive health care system in the world, spending more than \$4 trillion annually on health care.[1] Despite this exorbitant price tag and a complex network of private employer-sponsored and government-sponsored programs, nearly 10% of the US population lacks health insurance coverage.[2] Even among individuals with health insurance, fertility care is frequently excluded from covered services. Infertility affects 12% to 18% of US couples,[3,4] but the conditions have historically been viewed as a socially constructed disease and fertility treatments as "elective" interventions.[5] As a result, fertility care is predominantly paid for out-of-pocket (OOP) in the United States.

The lack of coverage for fertility care in the United States is largely out of touch with statements from national and international health care organizations as well as other developed countries. In 2009, the World Health Organization defined infertility as a disease,[6] and in 2015 the American Society of Reproductive medicine declared family

[a] Division of Reproductive Endocrinology and Infertility, Hospital of the University of Pennsylvania, 3701 Market Street, 8th Floor, Philadelphia, PA 19104, USA; [b] Department of Obstetrics & Gynecology, Duke University School of Medicine, 201 Trent Drive, 203 Baker House, Durham, NC 27710, USA; [c] Division of Reproductive Endocrinology & Infertility, Department of Obstetrics & Gynecology, Northwestern University Feinberg School of Medicine, 676 N. Saint Clair Street, Suite 2310, Chicago, IL 60611, USA
* Corresponding author. 676 N. Saint Clair Street, Suite 2310, Chicago, IL 60611.
E-mail address: tjain@northwestern.edu

Obstet Gynecol Clin N Am 50 (2023) 721–734
https://doi.org/10.1016/j.ogc.2023.08.002
0889-8545/23/© 2023 Elsevier Inc. All rights reserved.

obgyn.theclinics.com

building a basic human right.[7] Fourteen European countries provide full or partial coverage for in vitro fertilization (IVF),[8] the most effective treatment of infertility. Although 20 states now have legal mandates requiring payers to cover the diagnosis and/or treatment of infertility,[9] less than a third of all IVF cycles in the United States are performed in states with mandates that promote significant coverage of IVF.[10]

As with the overall American health care system, contradictions abound in the economics of fertility care. The US fertility industry results in net expenditures of approximately $2.4 billion each year,[11] but fewer than half of Americans with infertility have historically been able to access treatment.[12] Access to care is disproportionately low among low socioeconomic groups and certain racial and ethnic minorities.[13–17] Cost remains the greatest barrier to care for individuals,[18] but the proliferation of IVF "add-ons" such as preimplantation genetic testing (PGT) and intracytoplasmic sperm injection (ICSI) have contributed to rising per cycle costs in some settings.

In this review, the authors aim to describe the economics of fertility care in the United States, including the cost of IVF and IVF-associated technologies, insurance coverage for fertility care, and role of fertility care in addressing a declining world fertility rate and aging workforce and the increasing average age for family building. We hope that a better understanding of the economic issues shaping fertility can inform future policies aimed at promoting evidence-based practices and improving access to care in the United States.

THE COST OF INFERTILITY CARE

The estimated costs of fertility services vary widely. A summary of different fertility treatments and cost estimates are listed in **Table 1**. Ovulation induction (OI) is the least expensive form of fertility treatment of patients who do not spontaneously ovulate. Costs range from $25 to $242 with a single cycle of medications costing less than $10.[19–21] Cost effectiveness studies suggest that intrauterine insemination (IUI) ranges from $500 for OI + IUI to $2500 for a monitored, gonadotropin-based ovarian stimulation cycle with IUI.[22,23] IVF is the most effective and also most costly treatment of infertility. The American Society for Reproductive Medicine (ASRM) reports that the average cost of cycle of IVF is $12,400,[24] but this estimate has not been updated since it was first published in 2015. Other studies have suggested per cycle costs closer to $24,000.[25,26] A 2014 study by Wu and colleagues estimated that 18 months of IVF treatment costs on average $19,234 in terms of OOP expenditures.[21] Ultimately, a live birth is the most important outcome to patients struggling with infertility, but

Table 1 Cost of fertility treatments in the United States		
Treatment	**Cost ($)**	**Sources**
OI	$10–242	19–21
OI + IUI	$500	22,23
Gonadotropins + IUI + US monitoring	$2500	22,23
IVF	$12,400–24,000	24–26
Medications	$2000–6000	19,20
PGT-A	$1150–1650 per embryo	38–41
ICSI	$1500	30,51,52
Cost per live birth with IVF	~$70,000	26,27

Abbreviations: ICSI, intracytoplasmic sperm injection; IUI, intrauterine insemination; IVF, in vitro fertilization; OI, ovulation induction; PGT-A, preimplantation genetic testing for aneuploidy.

studies have estimated the cost per live birth with IVF can be more than $70,000 in 2021 US dollars.[26,27] Given the 2021 median household income in the United States was $70,784,[28] the average American would have to spend around a third of their annual income to afford a single cycle of IVF, or up to their entire annual earnings to achieve a live birth.

The difficulty with placing an exact price tag on infertility treatment stems from variations in treatment modalities, IVF protocols, and medication pricing based on brands and dosing. Patient-facing Web sites estimate that IVF medications alone add an additional $3000 to $6,000, gonadotropins heavily affecting this pricing.[19,20] Procedural costs play a significant role in the steep pricing. Egg retrieval has an estimated cost of $3922 with embryo cryopreservation adding an additional $800 to $1000 to the overall price without insurance coverage. Fresh embryo transfer is estimated to cost from $1050 to $1292, while frozen embryo transfer increases the price to a range of $3299 to $6906.[29] This does not include the price of ICSI, embryo biopsy, and preimplantation genetic testing for aneuploidy (PGT-A) testing which can drastically increase the overall OOP cost for the average patient. The procedural costs for OI by contrast are far lower with a monitored ovulation stimulation cycle estimated to cost $1754 for clinic and ultrasound fees based on one 2021 study.[29] IUIs can add an additional $300 to $800 to the overall price tag with a higher likelihood of insurance coverage compared with IVF.[20]

The excessive OOP burden for IVF has led Americans to go to drastic measures to afford fertility treatment. Although some clinics provide package pricing or repayment plans, many other families must turn to alternative means for payments. This can come in the form of personal or home equity loans, credit card charges, grants, and fundraising through crowdsource Web sites.[20,27,30] In 2021, Lai and colleagues reviewed crowdfunding campaigns over a 10 year period through GoFundMe, a popular crowdfunding Web site. They found that the average fertility treatment campaign goal was $18,639, but 77% of campaigns failed to meet their goal with campaigns averaging $6759 raised.[27]

With limited mechanisms for financial assistance, the economic burden of infertility treatment in the United States is the largest barrier to the access to care.[18,21] Without substantial changes in the cost of IVF or the degree of insurance coverage for fertility services in the United States, this unmet demand is unlikely to be met.

THE COST OF "ADD-ONS" TO IN VITRO FERTILIZATION: PREIMPLANTATION GENETIC TESTING FOR ANEUPLOIDY AND INTRACYTOPLASMIC SPERM INJECTION

Since the advent of IVF, additional technologies and techniques have arisen to be used in addition to traditional IVF; these assistive reproductive technology (ART) "add-ons" each claim to increase the likelihood of conception, implantation, or live birth. Many of these technologies were designed for specific etiologies of infertility or patient subpopulations, but over time have seen widespread use across all forms of infertility. For example, ICSI greatly improves the efficacy of IVF for couples with low sperm counts and quality, but today it has become standard of practice in many if not most IVF cycles,[31] despite recommendations by ASRM to avoid this practice.[32] Other "add-ons" include PGT-A,[33] endometrial receptivity assays, endometrial scratching, sperm DNA fragmentation analysis, and the in vitro maturation of oocytes. Each of these add-ons is debated in the literature with respect to each of their ultimate impact on outcomes; the cost effectiveness of these technologies can be even more controversial, if assessed at all. In the following section, we will look specifically at PGT-A and ICSI, the 2 most common infertility add-ons.

Preimplantation Genetic Testing for Aneuploidy

The goal of PGT-A is to screen embryos derived through IVF before embryo transfer and to increase meaningful implantation and live birth rates by selecting embryos with the highest likelihood to be euploid and therefore have greater odds of successful implantation and progression toward live birth. Overall, randomized controlled trials agree that PGT-A provides a meaningful increased likelihood of selecting embryos capable of sustaining long-term pregnancy and live birth among patients with recurrent pregnancy loss (RPL).[34–38] Furthermore, utilization of PGT-A in this population has the potential added benefit of reducing the number of resulting multiple gestation pregnancies (by facilitating utilization of single embryo transfer [SET]) and clinical miscarriages, each of which bear associated financial, time, and psychological costs.

Embryo biopsy and sequencing for PGT-A totals approximately $1150 to $1650 per embryo.[29,39–41] Several groups have directly questioned whether PGT-A is in fact cost effective. Collectively their results are divided but tend to agree that PGT-A may be cost effective in AMA and RPL populations, especially when primary goals include the reduction of time to live birth, and clinical miscarriages. Somigliana and colleagues came to this conclusion after a theoretic cost-effectiveness study wherein they compared SET of PGT-A selected embryos, versus serial SET of all available IVF-derived embryos. They found that cost-effectiveness is indeed increased when using PGT-A for patients of increasing age and number of available embryos.[42] Neal and colleagues came to similar conclusions after performing a decision analytical model of 74 IVF centers in New Jersey, describing that the use of PGT-A-selected embryos offered a cost-saving differential of $931 to $2411. These findings were driven by fewer transfers, cycles, and a reduction in the total time of treatment of aneuploid transfers and miscarriages.[39]

Conversely, PGT-A for younger patients, especially those less than 35 years of age, has not been shown to be cost effective. Collins and colleagues determined in their decision-analysis model that patient age must be 37 years or older to achieve a 4.2% increase in live birth rate at an additional cost of $4509. However, the incremental cost effectiveness ratio once at 37 years decreased costs from $145,063 per additional live birth using IVF, to $105,489 per live birth required to achieve a live birth using IVF without PGS.[43] In a similar criticism of PGT-A use for young patients, Scriven and colleagues showed that PGT-A significantly increases costs without improving live birth rate for most women under the age of 40 years.[44]

A recent analysis by Lee and colleagues developed a probabilistic decision tree and predicted the clinical costs from patient and societal perspectives.[38] The key difference between these perspectives was that patients were responsible for all IVF-related costs, whereas payers (and society at large) were additionally responsible for all obstetric costs related to prenatal care, miscarriage, and birth. From the patient perspective, the authors found that, for patients aged less than 35, no PGT-A was associated with lower incremental costs and higher live birth rates; after the age of 38 years, PGT-A was associated with lower costs and higher live birth rates. However, from a societal perspective, PGT-A was associated with lower incremental cost and cost per live birth due to lower rates of twin gestations and higher utilization of SET with PGT-A. Although younger individual patients lack an incentive to pursue PGT-A based on realized costs and worse outcomes, there may be justification for universal PGT-A from a societal perspective. As costs are likely to change over time along with associated technology improvements, such cost-effective analyses will need periodic reassessments.

Intracytoplasmic Sperm Injection

Since its invention in 1992 by Palermo and colleagues ICSI has seen a dramatic increase in utilization with IVF. Originally used only for severe male factor infertility, it now is frequently used for additional indications including advanced materal age (AMA), premature ovarian insufficiency (POI), idiopathic infertility, and the fertilization of previously frozen oocytes. In the United States, the proportion of IVF cycles utilizing ICSI increased from 11% in 1995 to 58% in 2004, more than quadrupling in 1 decade.[31] Despite this increase in frequency of use, published literature largely agrees that ICSI provides limited benefit in cases of non-male factor associated infertility,[45–47] with the exception of potential utility in cases of idiopathic fertilization failure after a first IVF cycle and auto-immune disease with anti-sperm antibodies.[48,49] Although the proportion of indicated cases for ICSI has remained relatively constant over the past few decades, the growth of ICSI suggests uptake in the absence of efficacy.[50] Nevertheless, ICSI has become incorporated into "standard" IVF protocol in many practices and laboratories.

ICSI adds approximately $1500 to an IVF cycle,[31,51,52] which adds substantial cost to an already costly procedure. In their Committee Opinion, ASRM only recommends ICSI for non-male factors infertility in selected patients undergoing IVF with PGT for monogenic conditions (to ensure monospermic fertilization and prevent contamination from extraneous, nonselected sperm) and with previously cryopreserved oocytes (given that cryopreservation may lead to changes to the zona pellucida that could reduce success with conventional fertilization).[32] Some authors have proposed that ICSI for non-male factor infertility only be used as a second line add-on, such as utilizing ICSI only after a primary IVF cycle has failed to achieve egg fertilization.[49]

The disproportionate utilization of PGT-A and ICSI in the absence of specific evidence or indications raises concerns regarding the future use of "add-ons" for IVF. Reproductive endocrinologists have been quick to adopt new technologies, optimistically due to a drive to innovate and improve patient outcomes. Furthermore, physicians may recommend additional treatments so that in the scenario where an IVF cycle is unsuccessful the physician can be seen to have done everything possible. Cynically, however, providers and practices may see novel "add-ons" as a means of differentiating themselves and generate additional profit margin in an increasingly competitive infertility marketplace. An increasing number of fertility practices are backed by private equity partners, which may further incentivize larger profits per patient. Although the motive is up for debate, "add-ons" for IVF will continue to proliferate if there is willingness to pay among patients and payers alike. In the absence of incentives and guidelines against their appropriate use, these "add-ons" are likely to continue to inflate the cost of IVF in the United States.

STATE INFERTILITY MANDATES

The number of IVF cycles performed in the United States has increased 153x over the past 3 decades, and in 2019, 2% of all infants born in the United States were the result of IVF.[53] Still, per capita IVF utilization in the United States pales in comparison to most European countries. In 2013, the European Society of Human Reproduction and Embryology estimated the population-based IVF demand to be 1500 cycles per million people.[54] Based on this calculation, the United States met only 67% of the presumed demand in 2019.[55,56]

State infertility insurance mandates are an essential component of expanding access to infertility services in the United States. Since 1977, 20 states have passed legislation requiring payers to cover services related to the diagnosis and management of infertility (**Fig. 1**).[5,9,57] However, these laws vary greatly in terms of patient

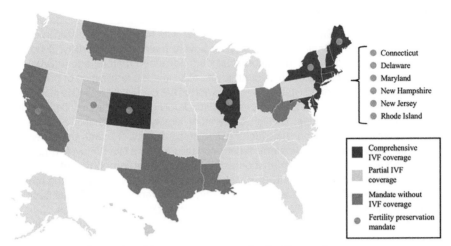

Fig. 1. States with mandated insurance coverage for fertility services.

eligibility, covered services, exclusions, and restrictions. Only 13 states currently mandate third party coverage for IVF, 11 of which (Connecticut, Colorado, Delaware, Illinois, Maine, Massachusetts, Maryland, New Hampshire, New Jersey, New York, and Rhode Island) provide "comprehensive" IVF coverage with minimal restrictions to patient eligibility, exemptions, and lifetime limits.[9]

Perhaps the most obvious impact of state infertility mandates is a resulting increase in utilization of fertility services. A recent retrospective analysis using 2018 data from the Centers for Disease Control and Prevention showed that states with comprehensive IVF mandates were associated with over double the per-capita nondonor IVF utilization compared with states without such mandates (6.2 vs 2.7 cycles per 1000 women ages 25–44 years).[10] These results make intuitive sense – as the OOP costs for IVF fall, more patients with infertility are able to afford treatment. This is consistent with economic models in the literature demonstrating that ART utilization increases by 3.2% for every 1% drop in costs in terms of disposable income.[25] Other studies have indicated that women with insurance coverage for IVF may be more likely to attempt additional IVF cycles following an initial unsuccessful cycle, resulting in a higher cumulative live birth rate compared with those women paying OOP for IVF.[58] Conversely, women without insurance coverage for IVF were more likely to discontinue treatment than those with insurance coverage.[59] A 2023 study using Society for Assisted Reproductive Technology (SART) data similarly found that IVF discontinuation rates were significantly higher in states without mandated insurance coverage.[60] In conjunction, these studies indicate that state infertility mandates covering IVF are associated with higher IVF utilization per capita and greater willingness to attempt multiple IVF cycles in the setting of a first unsuccessful cycle. As a result, one would expect significantly higher health care expenditures on infertility services in states with mandates. Unfortunately, no studies to-date have calculated this difference. However, a 2016 review of premium costs in Massachusetts following passage of their mandate showed that infertility treatments only accounted for 0.12% to 0.95% of premium costs statewide.[7]

Multiple studies have indicated that state infertility mandates are associated with differences in IVF practice patterns and outcomes. Elective single embryo transfer (eSET) is an increasingly common strategy used to reduce the risk of multiple gestations. Fertility treatments are responsible for one-third of all twin pregnancies and over three-quarters of triplet and higher order multiple pregnancies,[61] although it should be noted that non-IVF treatments have historically been responsible for a vast majority of higher order multiples.[62] Since the 2010s, several studies have noted higher rates of eSET utilization and resulting lower rates of multiples, especially among younger patients, in states with comprehensive IVF insurance mandates.[10,63–65] Economic modeling of ART affordability has supported this association, demonstrating that a 10% drop in the price of ART results in about a 5% increase in eSET utilization.[25] These differences in eSET and multiple births have significant maternal and neonatal consequences, as multiple births are associated with high rates of hypertensive disorders or pregnancy, gestational diabetes, preterm birth, hemorrhage, and stillbirth. These adverse outcomes are also significant associated with increased health care expenditures; according to one retrospective cohort study, twin and triplet deliveries cost 5x and 20x more than singleton pregnancies, respectively.[66] Recent data indicate that states with comprehensive IVF insurance mandates may also have higher live birth rates per cycle (35.4% vs 33.4%, $P = .03$), regardless of patient age.[10]

It is unclear whether the positive effects of mandates in terms of higher eSET, lower multiple births, and a higher live birth rate per cycle can offset the costs associated with increased utilization of IVF and lower treatment discontinuation rates. Additional research is needed to determine the added "value" of infertility treatments, both in terms of live births and reduced suffering by the afflicted patient and potential partner, as well as the potential impact of future mandates on state budgets and third-party payer health care expenditures.

EMPLOYER-SPONSORED INFERTILITY BENEFITS

Infertility coverage in the United States has increased as a part of employer-sponsored insurance plans over the past two decades. This reflects a positive shift in society's awareness of infertility, historically oversimplified and described as a social condition, and now more accurately understood to be a medical diagnosis deserving of high-quality health care and treatment. However, it also represents employers' understanding that infertility benefits could serve as a means of attracting and retaining reproductive age employees.

The costs of this to employers, and the potential economic, societal, and business incentives to increasing employer coverage of infertility is an increasingly popular point of interest and discussion. In an employer survey by Mercer in 2005, it was identified that 54% of employers with 500 employees or more covered infertility evaluation, and approximately 20% covered IVF.[67] In a case report of cost-effective infertility coverage, Southwest Airlines shared their experience of covering infertility care as defined by ASRM guidelines at facilities certified by the SART. Medical costs ranged from $126,000 to $188,000 per employee claim, yet costs across their study period represented less than 0.5% of their plan's total health care spending. This was markedly lower than expected, considering Southwest's workforce was predominantly of reproductive age.[68] Other reports from large employers indicated that a limited infertility benefit accounts for less than 0.5% to 0.8% of total health care expenditures.[68,69]

In a follow-up 2020 survey by Mercer of employer coverage for infertility, the percent of large companies providing coverage for the infertility work-up increased from 54% to 58%, with proportionally larger increases in coverage for IVF and oocyte cryopreservation (also known as fertility preservation), specifically. This trend was greatest among larger corporations with greater than 20,000 employees, among whom IVF coverage increased from 36% to 42%, and oocyte cryopreservation increased from 6% to 19%.[70] Interestingly, 97% of Mercer survey employer respondents who provided some form of infertility coverage to their employees endorsed a nonsignificant cost increase in their health plan expenditures. Among companies not presently providing infertility benefits, the leading attributed reason was a concern about associated costs; however, nearly half of these companies shared they would be more likely to provide infertility coverage if they knew costs would be offset, such as with decreased cases (and costs) due to multiple gestation pregnancies. One mechanism for preventing run-away spending on fertility treatments is through a lifetime benefit maximum. According to FertilityIQ, a patient-facing fertility education company, the average lifetime amount of fertility benefits covered among employees covered by a fertility benefit was $36,000 in 2021.[71] Although this number may be sufficient to cover a single IVF cycle, it may be insufficient for many patients to achieve a live birth.

Within the lay media, health care coverage for infertility has gathered a growing spotlight. With low unemployment and high job turnover post-COVID, increasing infertility coverage has become an important bargaining chip of successful companies to attract skilled employees and support social causes including diversity equity and inclusion. Some major companies, such as the ride-share company Lyft, are extending their coverage even further, including coverage for IVF, egg banking, surrogacy, and even adoption for groups that historically have not met criteria for a clinical infertility diagnosis (eg, LGTBQ + populations).[72] Leading the way in similar expansions of ART for family planning of its employees are Walmart and Amazon, the first and second largest employers in the United States, who also partner with infertility companies and benefit providers to expand their offered infertility services (eg, Amazon partnering with Progyny).[73] However, even though many of these large employers offer a fertility benefit, it does not mean that a majority of American employees have coverage. According to a 2022 Harris poll based on a survey of over 2000 US adults, only 6% of workers reported fertility benefit through their employer.[74] Many employees such as those who identify as LGBTQ + or single women may have a hard time accessing their employer's fertility benefit due to the heteronormative definition of infertility contained in many of these policies.

Infertility specialists and the general public both have been supportive of increasing employer-sponsored infertility benefits. A 2017 SART survey demonstrated that 78% of respondents supported insurance coverage of IVF for any clinical indication, with an even higher proportion of respondents supporting coverage for specific vulnerable populations, including patients with cancer (95%) and couples with life-altering inheritable genetic diseases (96%).[18] Similarly, in a 2021 survey sample of over 1000 US residents, a majority (55%) supported private insurance coverage of infertility services, including IVF.[75] Given this popular support and an increasingly competitive demand for workers in the setting of low unemployment, it is possible that market forces will continue to incentivize the proliferation of fertility benefits as an essential component of employer-sponsored health insurance. However, the private market is unlikely to make up for current disparities in access to fertility care, necessitating some degree of public policy to ensure reproductive justice for all populations, not just those working in highly competitive job markets.

DECLINING FERTILITY, ECONOMIC CONSEQUENCES, AND INFERTILITY CARE

Over the last half century from 1952 to 2022, the global fertility rate has declined approximately 50% and is continuing to fall.[76] The United States, among other developed nations, has not been immune to these global trends. Since 2007, birth rates in the United States have steadily declined and are predicted, along with fertility rates, to continue to decline.[77–79] Some high-income countries, such as Germany and Japan, have fertility rates that have fallen below 1.5 for the first time in over 20 years, which means women have had less than the necessary 2 children per women needed to maintain the present population size.[80]

Recently, the World Economic Forum proposed that this steady decline in fertility rates could have significant macroeconomic consequences. They suggest that if left without intervention, the declining fertility coupled with increasing life expectancy will result in a significantly older global population,[76] with the median age increasing from 25 year old in 1950 to 33 year old in 2020.[2] With fertility rates dropping below the replacement rate and a dramatically aging population, there is significant potential for economic consequences as a smaller workforce generates insufficient revenue to support programs such as Social Security and Medicare for a much larger generation of retirees than ever before.[80]

Naturally, other countries have become wary of this trend and have tested possible solutions to this problem or ways to help combat this declining fertility rate. Russia, France, and Sweden have implemented varying degrees of social benefits such as childcare services or tax breaks for larger families without much success in reversing a declining fertility rate.[81] In the United States, there has not been a unified policy approach to tackling this problem despite a clear need. As discussed elsewhere in this article, the utilization of IVF in the United States has increased dramatically over the past 40 years, with significantly 2 to 3x utilization among states with comprehensive IVF insurance mandates.[10] With infertility-associated costs accounting for less than 1% of total premium costs,[82] mandated insurance coverage of fertility care and IVF may be an effective strategy for combatting a declining fertility rate and the associated negative economic consequences. In support of this argument, one recent economics modeling study found that each child born from infertility treatment results in a 7-fold return in net-tax revenue.[83] As emphasized by the International Monetary Fund, covering of fertility services such as IVF and oocyte cryopreservation are an important part of supporting gender equality in the workplace.[80] Policies promoting coverage of infertility care could potentially increase fertility rates without compromising the increasing proportion of women joining and staying in the workforce.

It is important to acknowledge the limitations regarding the role of fertility care as a means of combating declining fertility rates and the associated economic consequences. It has yet to be seen if policies promoting fertility care have an ultimate effect large enough to combat formidable socioeconomic and cultural trends that have led to a declining fertility rate within developed economies. Given these shortcomings, advocates and policymakers should continue to look beyond the macroeconomic benefits when advocating for access to fertility care in the United States, invoking arguments such as treating infertility as a disease, addressing the psychosocial ills of infertility, and promoting gender equality and reproductive justice.

SUMMARY

Despite infertility being one of the most common medical conditions among reproductive-age populations, fertility treatments in the United States are expensive and cost prohibitive for most patients. Although the number of states with infertility insurance mandates has risen steadily in recent years, less than a quarter of IVF cycles in the United States are performed in states with a comprehensive IVF mandate.[10] Even though public and private insurers have the capacity to pay for IVF, many choose not to due to the historical perspective of considering infertility a social construct.

We hope this review draws attention to the economic challenges of providing high-quality care to Americans struggling with infertility. The field of reproductive endocrinology and infertility has demonstrated an immense capacity for innovation, but caution should be exercised when adopting new technologies to first ensure that they improve patient outcomes and result in cost-effective care. The concept of infertility as a social affliction not warranting the same coverage as other diseases is out of touch with the views of the public and medical community. Even though fertility benefits have gained cachet among employers as a means of attracting top talent, this trend is unlikely to result in equitable and widespread access to fertility care. The disparate coverage afforded by our fragmented health care system high-lights the importance of advocacy efforts to pass health care policies on a state and federal level to provide affordable fertility care for all in need.

DISCLOSURE

None.

REFERENCES

1. Centers for Medicare & Medicaid Services. National Healthcare Expenditure: Historical. Updated December 15, 2022, Available at: https://www.cms.gov/research-statistics-data-and-systems/statistics-trends-and-reports/nationalhealthexpenddata/nationalhealthaccountshistorical. Accessed February 9, 2023.
2. Cha AE, Cohen RA. Demographic Variation in Health Insurance Coverage:United States, 2021. Natl Health Stat Report 2022;(177):1–14.
3. Practice Committee of the American Society for Reproductive M. Diagnostic evaluation of the infertile female: a committee opinion. Fertil Steril 2015;103(6):e44–50.
4. Thoma ME, McLain AC, Louis JF, et al. Prevalence of infertility in the United States as estimated by the current duration approach and a traditional constructed approach. Fertil Steril 2013;99(5):1324–31.e1.
5. Kawwass JF, Penzias AS, Adashi EY. Fertility-a human right worthy of mandated insurance coverage: the evolution, limitations, and future of access to care. Fertil Steril 2021;115(1):29–42.
6. Zegers-Hochschild F, Adamson GD, de Mouzon J, et al. International Committee for Monitoring Assisted Reproductive Technology (ICMART) and the World Health Organization (WHO) revised glossary of ART terminology, 2009. Fertil Steril 2009;92(5):1520–4.
7. Ethics Committee of the American Society for Reproductive Medicine. Disparities in access to effective treatment for infertility in the United States: an Ethics Committee opinion. Fertil Steril 2021;116(1):54–63.
8. Berg Brigham K, Cadier B, Chevreul K. The diversity of regulation and public financing of IVF in Europe and its impact on utilization. Hum Reprod 2013;28(3):666–75.
9. Peipert BJ, Montoya MN, Bedrick BS, et al. Impact of in vitro fertilization state mandates for third party insurance coverage in the United States: a review and critical assessment. Reprod Biol Endocrinol 2022;20(1):111.
10. Peipert BJ, Chung EH, Harris BS, et al. Impact of comprehensive state insurance mandates on in vitro fertilization utilization, embryo transfer practices, and outcomes in the United States. Am J Obstet Gynecol 2022. https://doi.org/10.1016/j.ajog.2022.03.003.
11. Kennedy K. OD4036: Fertility Clinics. IBIS World. Updated 2/2/2020, Available at: https://my.ibisworld.com/us/en/industry-specialized/od4036/. Accessed July 5, 2020.

12. Chambers GM, Sullivan EA, Ishihara O, et al. The economic impact of assisted reproductive technology: a review of selected developed countries. Fertil Steril 2009;91(6):2281–94.
13. Jain T, Hornstein MD. Disparities in access to infertility services in a state with mandated insurance coverage. Fertil Steril 2005;84(1):221–3.
14. Jain T. Socioeconomic and racial disparities among infertility patients seeking care. Fertil Steril 2006;85(4):876–81.
15. Galic I, Negris O, Warren C, et al. Disparities in access to fertility care: who's in and who's out. F S Rep 2021;2(1):109–17.
16. Komorowski AS, Jain T. A review of disparities in access to infertility care and treatment outcomes among Hispanic women. Reprod Biol Endocrinol 2022; 20(1):1.
17. Seifer DB, Sharara FI, Jain T. The Disparities in ART (DART) Hypothesis of Racial and Ethnic Disparities in Access and Outcomes of IVF Treatment in the USA. Reprod Sci 2022. https://doi.org/10.1007/s43032-022-00888-0.
18. Seifer DB, Wantman E, Sparks AE, et al. National survey of the Society for Assisted Reproductive Technology membership regarding insurance coverage for assisted reproductive technologies. Fertil Steril 2018;110(6):1081–1088 e1.
19. Li D. How Much Do IVF (In Vitro Fertilization) Medications Cost? GoodRx.com, Available at: https://www.goodrx.com/health-topic/parenthood-pregnancy/ivf-in-vitro-fertilization-medications-cost. Accessed February 9, 2023.
20. Conrad M, Whitfield, J. A Beginner's Guide To Fertility Treatments. Forbes.com. Updated Jun 15, 2022, Available at: https://www.forbes.com/health/family/fertility-treatments-guide/. Accessed February 9, 2023.
21. Wu AK, Odisho AY, Washington SL 3rd, et al. Out-of-pocket fertility patient expense: data from a multicenter prospective infertility cohort. J Urol 2014; 191(2):427–32.
22. Reindollar RH, Regan MM, Neumann PJ, et al. A randomized clinical trial to evaluate optimal treatment for unexplained infertility: the fast track and standard treatment (FASTT) trial. Fertil Steril 2010;94(3):888–99.
23. Yu B, Mumford S, Royster GDt, et al. Cost-effectiveness analysis comparing continuation of assisted reproductive technology with conversion to intrauterine insemination in patients with low follicle numbers. Fertil Steril 2014;102(2):435–9.
24. American Society of Reproductive Medicine. WHITEPAPER: Access to Care Summit. presented at: ASRM Access to Care Summit; September 10-11, 2015 2015; Washington, DC.
25. Chambers GM, Hoang VP, Sullivan EA, et al. The impact of consumer affordability on access to assisted reproductive technologies and embryo transfer practices: an international analysis. Fertil Steril 2014;101(1):191–198 e4.
26. Katz P, Showstack J, Smith JF, et al. Costs of infertility treatment: results from an 18-month prospective cohort study. Fertil Steril 2011;95(3):915–21.
27. Lai JD, Fantus RJ, Cohen AJ, et al. Unmet financial burden of infertility care and the impact of state insurance mandates in the United States: analysis from a popular crowdfunding platform. Fertil Steril 2021. https://doi.org/10.1016/j.fertnstert.2021.05.111.
28. Semega J, Kollar, M. Income in the United States: 2021. 2022. September 13, 2022. Available at: https://www.census.gov/library/publications/2022/demo/p60-276.html. Accessed February 9, 2023.
29. Lee M, Lofgren KT, Thomas A, et al. The cost-effectiveness of preimplantation genetic testing for aneuploidy in the United States: an analysis of cost and birth

outcomes from 158,665 in vitro fertilization cycles. Am J Obstet Gynecol 2021; 225(1):55 e1–e55 e17.

30. Peipert BJ, Hairston JC, McQueen DB, et al. Increasing access to fertility care through private foundations. Fertil Steril 2019;111(6):1211–6.

31. Jain T, Gupta RS. Trends in the use of intracytoplasmic sperm injection in the United States. N Engl J Med 2007;357(3):251–7.

32. Practice Committees of the American Society for Reproductive M, the Society for Assisted Reproductive Technology. Electronic address aao. Intracytoplasmic sperm injection (ICSI) for non-male factor indications: a committee opinion. Fertil Steril 2020;114(2):239–45.

33. Bedrick BS, Tipping AD, Nickel KB, et al. State-Mandated Insurance Coverage and Preimplantation Genetic Testing in the United States. Obstet Gynecol 2022;139(4):500–8.

34. Scott RT Jr, Upham KM, Forman EJ, et al. Blastocyst biopsy with comprehensive chromosome screening and fresh embryo transfer significantly increases in vitro fertilization implantation and delivery rates: a randomized controlled trial. Fertil Steril 2013;100(3):697–703.

35. Verpoest W, Staessen C, Bossuyt PM, et al. Preimplantation genetic testing for aneuploidy by microarray analysis of polar bodies in advanced maternal age: a randomized clinical trial. Hum Reprod 2018;33(9):1767–76.

36. Munne S, Kaplan B, Frattarelli JL, et al. Preimplantation genetic testing for aneuploidy versus morphology as selection criteria for single frozen-thawed embryo transfer in good-prognosis patients: a multicenter randomized clinical trial. Fertil Steril 2019;112(6):1071–1079 e7.

37. Bhatt SJ, Marchetto NM, Roy J, et al. Pregnancy outcomes following in vitro fertilization frozen embryo transfer (IVF-FET) with or without preimplantation genetic testing for aneuploidy (PGT-A) in women with recurrent pregnancy loss (RPL): a SART-CORS study. Hum Reprod 2021;36(8):2339–44.

38. Sato T, Sugiura-Ogasawara M, Ozawa F, et al. Preimplantation genetic testing for aneuploidy: a comparison of live birth rates in patients with recurrent pregnancy loss due to embryonic aneuploidy or recurrent implantation failure. Hum Reprod 2019;34(12):2340–8.

39. Neal SA, Morin SJ, Franasiak JM, et al. Preimplantation genetic testing for aneuploidy is cost-effective, shortens treatment time, and reduces the risk of failed embryo transfer and clinical miscarriage. Fertil Steril 2018;110(5):896–904.

40. Goldman RH, Racowsky C, Farland LV, et al. The cost of a euploid embryo identified from preimplantation genetic testing for aneuploidy (PGT-A): a counseling tool. J Assist Reprod Genet 2018;35(9):1641–50.

41. Mersereau JE, Plunkett BA, Cedars MI. Preimplantation genetic screening in older women: a cost-effectiveness analysis. Fertil Steril 2008;90(3):592–8.

42. Somigliana E, Busnelli A, Paffoni A, et al. Cost-effectiveness of preimplantation genetic testing for aneuploidies. Fertil Steril 2019;111(6):1169–76.

43. Collins SC, Xu X, Mak W. Cost-effectiveness of preimplantation genetic screening for women older than 37 undergoing in vitro fertilization. J Assist Reprod Genet 2017;34(11):1515–22.

44. Scriven PN. Towards a better understanding of preimplantation genetic screening for aneuploidy: insights from a virtual trial for women under the age of 40 when transferring embryos one at a time. Reprod Biol Endocrinol 2017;15(1):49.

45. Geng T, Cheng L, Ge C, et al. The effect of ICSI in infertility couples with non-male factor: a systematic review and meta-analysis. J Assist Reprod Genet 2020; 37(12):2929–45.

46. Bosch E, Espinos JJ, Fabregues F, et al. ALWAYS ICSI? A SWOT analysis. J Assist Reprod Genet 2020;37(9):2081–92.

47. Zhang L, Cai H, Li W, et al. Duration of infertility and assisted reproductive outcomes in non-male factor infertility: can use of ICSI turn the tide? BMC Wom Health 2022;22(1):480.

48. van der Westerlaken L, Helmerhorst F, Dieben S, et al. Intracytoplasmic sperm injection as a treatment for unexplained total fertilization failure or low fertilization after conventional in vitro fertilization. Fertil Steril 2005;83(3):612–7.

49. Balli M, Cecchele A, Pisaturo V, et al. Opportunities and Limits of Conventional IVF versus ICSI: It Is Time to Come off the Fence. J Clin Med 2022;11(19). https://doi.org/10.3390/jcm11195722.

50. Boulet SL, Mehta A, Kissin DM, et al. Trends in use of and reproductive outcomes associated with intracytoplasmic sperm injection. JAMA 2015;313(3):255–63.

51. Dieke AC, Mehta A, Kissin DM, et al. Intracytoplasmic sperm injection use in states with and without insurance coverage mandates for infertility treatment, United States, 2000-2015. Fertil Steril 2018;109(4):691–7.

52. Iwamoto A, Van Voorhis BJ, Summers KM, et al. Intracytoplasmic sperm injection vs. conventional in vitro fertilization in patients with non-male factor infertility. Fertil Steril 2022;118(3):465–72.

53. Sunderam S, Kissin DM, Zhang Y, et al. Assisted Reproductive Technology Surveillance - United States, 2017. MMWR Surveill Summ 2020;69(9):1–20.

54. Group ECW. Social determinants of human reproduction. Hum Reprod 2001; 16(7):1518–26.

55. Centers for Disease Control and Prevention. 2019 Assisted Reproductive Technology Fertility Clinic and National Summary Report. 2021. Available at: https://www.cdc.gov/art/reports/2019/pdf/2019-Report-ART-Fertility-Clinic-National-Summary-h.pdf. Accessed March 1, 2023.

56. United States Census Bureau. QuickFacts: United States, 2020. Available at: www.census.gov/quickfacts/fact/table/US/PST045219. Accessed March 1, 2023.

57. RESOLVE: The National Infertility Association. Infertility Coverage By State. Updated June 2022, Available at: https://resolve.org/what-are-my-options/insurance-coverage/infertility-coverage-state/. Accessed February 22, 2023.

58. Jungheim ES, Leung MY, Macones GA, et al. In Vitro Fertilization Insurance Coverage and Chances of a Live Birth. JAMA 2017;317(12):1273–5.

59. Bedrick BS, Anderson K, Broughton DE, et al. Factors associated with early in vitro fertilization treatment discontinuation. Fertil Steril 2019;112(1):105–11.

60. Lee JC, DeSantis CE, Yartel AK, et al. Association of state insurance coverage mandates with assisted reproductive technology care discontinuation. Am J Obstet Gynecol 2023;228(3):315.e1-14.

61. Kulkarni AD, Adashi EY, Jamieson DJ, et al. Affordability of Fertility Treatments and Multiple Births in the United States. Paediatr Perinat Epidemiol 2017;31(5):438–48.

62. Kulkarni AD, Jamieson DJ, Jones HW Jr, et al. Fertility treatments and multiple births in the United States. N Engl J Med 2013;369(23):2218–25.

63. Provost MP, Thomas SM, Yeh JS, et al. State Insurance Mandates and Multiple Birth Rates After In Vitro Fertilization. Obstet Gynecol 2016;128(6):1205–14.

64. Jain T, Harlow BL, Hornstein MD. Insurance coverage and outcomes of in vitro fertilization. N Engl J Med 2002;347(9):661–6.

65. Crawford S, Boulet SL, Jamieson DJ, et al. Assisted reproductive technology use, embryo transfer practices, and birth outcomes after infertility insurance mandates: New Jersey and Connecticut. Fertil Steril 2016;105(2):347–55.

66. Lemos EV, Zhang D, Van Voorhis BJ, et al. Healthcare expenses associated with multiple vs singleton pregnancies in the United States. Am J Obstet Gynecol 2013;209(6):586 e1–e586 e11.

67. Mercer Health & Benefits. Employer experience with, and attitudes toward, coverage of infertility treatment. 2006. Available at: http://familybuilding.resolve.org/site/DocServer/Mercer_-_Resolve_Final_report.pdf?docID=4361. Accessed February 25, 2023.

68. Silverberg K, Meletiche D, Del Rosario G. An employer's experience with infertility coverage: a case study. Fertil Steril 2009;92(6):2103–5.

69. Van Voorhis BJ, Stovall DW, Allen BD, et al. Cost-effective treatment of the infertile couple. Fertil Steril 1998;70(6):995–1005.

70. Mercer LLC. 2021 Survey on Fertility Benefits. 2021. Available at: https://resolve.org/wp-content/uploads/2022/01/2021-Fertility-Survey-Report-Final.pdf. Accessed February 24, 2023.

71. FertilityIQ. 2021 FertilityIQ Workplace Index. FertilityIQ.com, Available at: https://www.fertilityiq.com/topics/fertilityiq-data-and-notes/fertilityiq-workplace-index. Accessed February 22, 2023.

72. Cerullo M. The latest employee benefit? Helping workers have babies. CBS News, 2022. Available at: https://www.cbsnews.com/news/fertility-reproductive-benefits-important-for-recruitment-inclusion/

73. Gonzales O, Dreher A. Employers expand reproductive health benefits amid tight labor market. Axios. October 11, 2022. Available at: https://www.axios.com/2022/10/11/fertility-benefit-reproductive-health-labor. Accessed March 1, 2023.

74. Leonhardt M. Fertility benefits have become a major weapon in the war for talent. Fortune. Accessed February 22, 2023, Available at: https://fortune.com/2022/03/05/fertility-benefits-are-a-major-weapon-in-the-war-for-talent/

75. Ho JR, Aghajanova L, Mok-Lin E, et al. Public attitudes in the United States toward insurance coverage for in vitro fertilization and the provision of infertility services to lower income patients. F&S Reports 2021. https://doi.org/10.1016/j.xfre.2021.09.002.

76. Pablo Alvarez. What does the global decline of the fertility rate look like? World Economic Forum, Available at: https://www.weforum.org/agenda/2022/06/global-decline-of-fertility-rates-visualised/. Accessed February 25, 2023.

77. Martin JA, Hamilton BE, Osterman MJ, et al. Births: final data for 2013. Natl Vital Stat Rep 2015;64(1):1–65.

78. Martin JA, Hamilton BE, Osterman MJK, et al. Births: Final Data for 2018. Natl Vital Stat Rep 2019;68(13):1–47.

79. Martin JA, Hamilton BE, Osterman MJK, et al. Births: Final Data for 2019. Natl Vital Stat Rep 2021;70(2):1–51.

80. Doepke M, Hannusch A, Kindermann F, Tertilt M. The New Economics of Fertility 2022. Finance & Development. Available at: https://www.imf.org/en/Publications/fandd/issues/Series/Analytical-Series/new-economics-of-fertility-doepke-hannusch-kindermann-tertilt. Accessed February 25, 2023.

81. BBC News. How do countries fight falling birth rates? BBC News. Available at: https://www.bbc.com/news/world-europe-51118616. Accessed March 1, 2023.

82. Weigel G, Ranji U, Long M, Salganicoff A. Coverage and Use of Fertility Services in the U.S. Kaiser Family Foundation, Available at: https://www.kff.org/womens-health-policy/issue-brief/coverage-and-use-of-fertility-services-in-the-u-s/. Accessed February 22, 2023.

83. Connolly MP, Kotsopoulos N, Eisenberg ML. The intergenerational economics of infertility, childrearing, and assisted reproduction. Fertil Steril 2023;119(2):184–5.

Breaking Down Barriers
Advancing Toward Health Equity in Fertility Care for Black and Hispanic Patients

Aileen Portugal, MD[a,b], Alyssa K. Kosturakis, MD, MS[c],
Ticara L. Onyewuenyi, MD, MPH[d], Greysha Rivera-Cruz, MD[e],
Patricia T. Jimenez, MD[b,*]

KEYWORDS

- Fertility • Health disparities • Health equity

KEY POINTS

- Infertility can affect all people, regardless of race, ethnicity, or socioeconomic status.
- Barriers to quality fertility care include access, financial limitations, education, and social stigmas.
- Although racial disparities in outcomes of assisted reproductive technology can be largely attributed to the impacts of systemic racism (not race), we can make changes to improve equity of care.
- We propose strategies in the areas of advocacy, clinical setting, community, and outcomes to address the racial disparities.

BACKGROUND

Around 6.7 million women in the United States experience infertility.[1] According to the National Health and Nutrition Examination Survey data from 2013 through 2016, infertility rates did not differ by race or ethnicity.[2] However, compared with White patients, Black and Hispanic patients are less likely to receive infertility treatments, have lower clinical intrauterine pregnancy rates, lower live birth rates, and higher rates of spontaneous abortions.[3,4] To begin to reduce these racial disparities, the American Society

[a] Department of Obstetrics, Gynecology, University of California San Francisco, 490 Illinois Street, 10th Floor, Box 0132, San Francisco, CA 94158, USA; [b] Department of Obstetrics and Gynecology, Division of Reproductive Endocrinology and Infertility, Washington University, 4444 Forest Park Avenue, Ste. 3100, St. Louis, MO 63108, USA; [c] Department of Obstetrics and Gynecology, University of Washington, 1959 NE Pacific Street, Box 356460, Seattle, WA 98195-6460, USA; [d] Department of Obstetrics and Gynecology, Kaiser Permanente Northern California, 3600 Broadway, Oakland, CA 94611, USA; [e] Herbert Wertheim College Medicine, Florida International University, 3251 North State Road 7 Suite 200, Margate, FL 33063, USA
* Corresponding author.
E-mail address: jimenezp@wustl.edu

Obstet Gynecol Clin N Am 50 (2023) 735–746
https://doi.org/10.1016/j.ogc.2023.08.007
0889-8545/23/© 2023 Elsevier Inc. All rights reserved.

for Reproductive Medicine (ASRM) added "access to care" as a key area of focus in its 2014 to 2019 strategic plan. This included emphasizing research and advocacy to identify and address racial disparities.[5] In 2020, ASRM reaffirmed its commitment by creating a Task Force on Diversity, Equity, and Inclusion with the goal of reducing and ultimately eliminating health disparities in access and outcomes to reproductive care. This review summarizes the research on the nature of racial disparities in fertility care. It also discusses strategies to improve reproductive health-care access and outcomes for Black and Hispanic patients.

Access to Care

Socioeconomic barriers

A key barrier to accessing infertility care is the high cost of treatments, which may not be covered by insurance and can be inaccessible to people with lower incomes. According to ASRM, the average cost of an in vitro fertilization (IVF) cycle with medications is US$19,200.[6] This cost may be more affordable for non-Hispanic White families, whose median household income in 2021 was US$74,262, than for non-Hispanic Black or Hispanic families, who had median incomes of US$48,297 and US$57,981,[7] respectively. Unfortunately, even when the cost of infertility care is mitigated, Black and Hispanic patients still face barriers to infertility care. For example, Massachusetts mandates insurance coverage for infertility, which would level the field if cost were the only factor. However, although 6.8% of the state population is Hispanic, only 3.9% of infertility patients are Hispanic.[8,9] Similar disparities were observed in the military health-care system. Whereas 9% of personnel in the Department of Defense are Hispanic, only 4% of patients seeking infertility treatment are Hispanic.[10] Furthermore, although about 12.5% of the US population is Hispanic, only 5.4% of the assisted reproductive technology (ART) population is Hispanic.[11] Although a 2022 study showed that the utilization rate of IVF was higher for all women in states with insurance mandates than in states without an insurance mandate,[10] the greatest difference was among White and Asian women.[12] Thus, although insurance mandates increased access for some women, the racial disparities persist[12,13] suggesting that factors other than cost affect minority patients' access to ART.

Education and knowledge barriers

A second potential barrier to equitable fertility care is reproductive health literacy, defined as an individual's "capacity to obtain, process and understand basic health information and services needed to make appropriate health decisions."[14,15] Several investigators have evaluated fertility awareness and found that, among people of reproductive age, fertility awareness is generally low. People seem to be familiar with infertility as an issue and the majority can understand basic age-related changes. In a study by Meissner and colleagues, almost 80% of the college students surveyed were aware that women's fertility starts to decline in the 30s. However, the vast majority of these students overestimated fecundability for a couple in their 20s.[16] Nevertheless, there is still limited understanding of age-related changes, male risk factors, spontaneous pregnancy rates, and fertility treatments.[17]

This lack of reproductive literacy is especially prevalent among patients with low socio-economic status and level of education.[18] Moreover, Black and Hispanic women seem to have lower fertility awareness than White women.[19] This is important because fertility knowledge is positively associated with shorter time to seek fertility evaluation and treatment,[20] and the sooner a person seeks treatment, the better their chance of becoming pregnant. In a survey study, Insogna and colleagues reported that Hispanic and Black or African American women had longer delays in presenting for fertility evaluation compared with White women. Specifically, at 12 months of trying to conceive, 65% of Hispanic women, 47% of Black women, and 78% of White women sought care.[21] Low-resource Hispanic patients seem especially vulnerable because they have lower fertility awareness than high-resource nonimmigrant patients.[18] Maher and colleagues explored the associations between race and subfertility risk factors. Hispanic women were less likely than White women to recognize the effects of smoking on fertility, whereas Black patients tended to acknowledge the relationship between sexually transmitted infections and infertility.[22] However, this study was limited by the small representation of Black and Hispanic patients among the study groups. In a study examining reproductive health literacy, 46% of Black women from an urban clinic correctly understood the relationship between body mass index and fertility but only 24% understood that fertility decreases with age.[23] Given these findings, we must improve reproductive health literacy to reduce disparities in access to and utilization of reproductive health services.

Social stigma

A third potential barrier to reproductive health equity is social stigma. In many communities, infertility can be considered a taboo topic of discussion and may be seen as a personal failure or a source of shame. For example, one fertility clinic-based questionnaire of 743 women seeking infertility care showed that Black women were more likely than White women to report that they were concerned about social stigmatization and disappointing a spouse because of their infertility.[24] Black women also were more likely than White women to report concern about friends and family finding out about treatment and to self-refer for care, suggesting a lack of support for care seeking for infertility in their social network. Another study in which Hispanic women were interviewed revealed a recurring belief that children were the basis of the marital relationship and that childless marriages were considered a failure.[25] As a result of social stigmas, Black and Hispanic women may be hesitant to seek help or talk about their experiences, making it difficult for them to access information about fertility options and find support from friends and family. This stigmatization may cause couples to delay or avoid seeking treatment.

Black patients are often stigmatized by the harmful stereotype that Black women are inherently more fertile than women of other races. This "Black fertility myth," a term coined by Dr Tia Jackson-Bey, is rooted in racist beliefs that can be dated back to the era of slavery.[23] Although this myth has been disproven by multiple studies showing that Black women experience infertility at rates similar to those of other races,[2,19,26,27] it has been used to deny Black women access to fertility care and resources. Furthermore, it implies that Black women's reproductive decisions are not valuable and can be ignored. Unfortunately, this false stereotype persists in many Black communities, leading to personal shame and delay in seeking fertility care.[23,24] Whether similar stereotypes or assumptions exist about the fertility of Hispanic individuals is unclear but should be considered as we seek ways to reduce disparities in health-care access.

Outcomes

Unfortunately, once Black and Hispanic patients with infertility overcome the barriers to receiving care, they often experience disparities in ART outcomes. For example, Seifer and colleagues showed, compared with White patients, African Americans were 30% less likely to achieve a live birth in 1999 to 2000 and 36% less likely in 2015 to 2016.[28] In one study, early pregnancy loss after IVF was higher in Black women than White women (8.0% vs 6.9%, $P = .018$).[22] In a different population, McQueen and colleagues reported that the spontaneous abortion rate after IVF was 28.9% in Black women and 14.6% in White women[3]. Black and Hispanic women also have higher odds of adverse pregnancy outcomes such as fetal growth restriction and preterm delivery when compared with White women.[29] A systematic review showed that White women consistently had the highest rates of live births when compared with Black and Hispanic women,[30] suggesting significant racial disparities in IVF outcomes in the United States.

Several factors may contribute to the disparity in outcomes for Black women, most of which can be traced to systemic racism and the overall health inequities in the United States. First, likely because of delays in seeking care and referral patterns, Black women tend to be at an older age when seeking fertility treatment than White women. For example, Ghidei and colleagues showed that Black patients seeking fertility care were significantly more likely than White patients to be aged greater than 35 years (61% vs 50%, $P < .01$).[31] On average, Black and Hispanic women have been attempting to conceive for 1.5 years longer than White women at initial fertility evaluation.[24,32] This delay in accessing care can have detrimental long-term impacts on treatment outcomes because increased duration of infertility before seeking treatment is a poor prognostic indicator of treatment success.[31] Black women have other factors that affect fertility treatment success and pregnancy outcomes. Compared with White women, they have higher body mass index, are 3 times more likely to have diabetes, have a 2-fold greater risk of spontaneous abortions, and are 3 times more likely to have leiomyomas.[3,11,31]

Hispanic populations also experience disparities in ART outcomes. For example, national data from the Society for Assisted Reproductive Technology (SART) Writing Group 2010 demonstrated that Hispanic women receiving ART were 13% less likely than White women to achieve a live birth.[11] Similarly, in a retrospective cohort study from the Society for Assisted Reproductive Technology Clinic Outcome Reporting System (SARTCORS) database for 2014 to 2016, Kotlyar and colleagues demonstrated that Hispanic women had a lower cumulative live birth rate than White women (OR 0.84, 95% CI: 0.77–0.92).[33] Multiple approaches will likely be needed to reduce these disparities in outcomes.

Lack of Diversity Within the Specialty

One potential strategy to improve outcomes for Black and Hispanic patients undergoing infertility treatment is to increase the diversity of providers. Many studies suggest positive patient perception and improved patient outcomes when patients identify ethnically and racially with their providers; however, others show no difference in patient satisfaction when patient–provider dyads are similar.[34–41]

Reproductive endocrinology and infertility (REI) specialists are predominantly White, and this fact is not likely to change soon. This is because an analysis of REI trainees in 2018 showed that, of 156 clinical fellows, 11 (7%) identified as Black, 0 (0%) identified as American Indian or Native Hawaiian/Pacific Islander, and 5 (3%) identified as Hispanic or Latino.[42] These numbers are far less than the national population; in 2021, 12.6% of people in the United States were Black, 0.9% were American Indian or Native Hawaiian/Pacific Islander, and 18.9% were Hispanic or Latino.[34] Given the small numbers of minority REI physicians and minority patients receiving infertility care, no studies exist in the infertility literature regarding patient–physician racial concordance. However, a few studies from other health-care specialties may provide insight.

First, in a telephone survey of patients with appointments at multiple primary care practices, patients in race–concordant relationships with their physicians rated their visits as significantly more "participatory" and were more satisfied with their care than patients in race–discordant relationships.[35] Second, in a study examining post-partum patients, there was no difference in perceptions of intrapartum care between racially concordant and discordant physician–patient dyads. However, this study was underpowered to detect a difference in the participant assessment of discrimination they faced due to race or ethnicity.[36] Third, in a large cross-sectional study including 92,238 patients and 747 physicians across 4 racial/ethnic groups (White, Black, Asian, and Hispanic) and male or female gender, patients rated the likelihood of recommending their physician to others on a numerical scale. Black patients were more likely to assign lower ratings to White physicians. However, this study was limited by the overall high socioeconomic status of those surveyed, which fails to capture the experience of the most vulnerable subset of patients.[37,38] Finally, a randomized trial assigned participants video vignettes of physicians and requested ratings based on predefined characteristics. Black patients viewed Black physicians more positively and were more receptive to the same medical recommendation when delivered by a Black physician than when delivered by a White physician.[39]

Several review articles discuss patient–provider race concordance. One review of 27 published studies from 1980 to 2008 noted that 33% of studies reported an association between patient–provider race concordance and positive health outcomes for minorities, 30% reported no association, and 37% reported mixed associations.[40] Another review article reports similarly inconclusive findings.[41] These studies highlight the complex nature of the patient–provider relationship, which is modified significantly by many other factors, including gender concordance, primary language concordance, education, and length of relationship with provider. Therefore, although race concordance may be a primary predictor of perceived similarity, several factors can affect perceived patient–provider similarity, including gender, personal beliefs, and personal values. These intangible characteristics combine with provider race to affect patient satisfaction, trust, and adherence to treatment.[43]

A PROPOSED STRATEGY TO REDUCE DISPARITIES IN FERTILITY CARE

To help dismantle the disparities in fertility care and improve outcomes, we propose a novel framework of strategies in 4 areas: advocacy, clinical setting, community, and outcomes (**Fig. 1**).

Advocacy

We propose several potential advocacy goals to increase equitable infertility care. First, truly universal health insurance coverage for fertility care, without exceptions and exclusions, is necessary to improve access and reduce disparities. In 2021, only 14 states in the US mandate insurers to cover infertility care.[44] These mandates are one of 2 types. "Mandated coverage" laws require health insurance companies to provide coverage of infertility treatment as a benefit in every policy. "Mandated to offer" law requires health insurance companies to make available for purchase a policy that offers coverage of infertility treatment.[45] Massachusetts is often cited as the gold standard for infertility insurance coverage. However, Koniares and colleagues revealed that the Massachusetts Infertility Insurance Mandate grants exemptions to Medicare, MassHealth, TRICARE, and self-insured companies.[9] As a result, only between 26.2% and 36.0% of reproductive-age women in Massachusetts are eligible for infertility coverage.[8] Massachusetts is not alone in this fact because most states that mandate coverage also have exclusions or exceptions to the law that limits patients' access to that coverage.

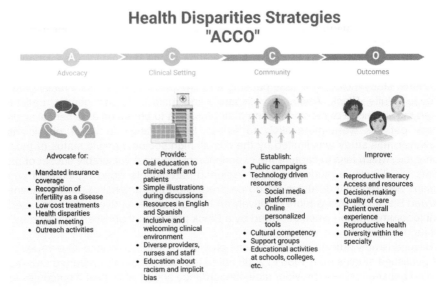

Fig. 1. Proposed strategies to reduce racial disparities in fertility care. (Created with BioRender.com.)

Second, ART providers can promote the fact that infertility is defined as a disease by the World Health Organization, the American Medical Association, and the ASRM. Such promotion may increase insurance coverage and reduce the social stigma surrounding infertility in some communities.

Third, strategies to increase the physical reach of fertility care are required. For instance, one study showed that minority women traveled twice the distance as White women to receive care at a fertility clinic.[46] The authors suggest that minority women more frequently live in neighborhoods with fewer resources overall, including fewer medical facilities.[46] In addition to establishing fertility clinics in low-income and middle-income communities, developing low-cost IVF options may help increase access. One such innovative option is "Invocell" a novel intravaginal culture device designed to provide a natural fertilization environment. Further research is needed to develop methods and devices with comparable pregnancy outcomes as traditional IVF. We are optimistic that the "femtech" arena will yield new advances to reduce the cost of ART and make it accessible to more patients.

Fourth, annual meetings focused on health disparities in fertility care should be held at the local and national levels. Conferences can focus on the latest research on health disparities, current initiatives aimed at reducing these disparities, and best practices for improving access to fertility care for underserved communities. The meetings may provide a space for community members to share their experiences and provide feedback on existing initiatives, helping clinics to better tailor their efforts to meet the needs of the community. Organizations must demonstrate a commitment to promoting diversity, equity, inclusion, and accountability to the wider community in their efforts to reduce health disparities in fertility care.

Fifth, to address the lack of fertility knowledge and awareness of available options among Black and Hispanic populations, ART providers can increase education and outreach initiatives. Potential initiatives include culturally sensitive and language-specific educational materials, community outreach programs, and partnerships with local organizations to provide information and resources on fertility options. Greater accessibility via telemedicine and online resources may increase access to care. Together, these efforts may reduce the barriers to fertility care and increase the utilization of these services among these communities.

Clinical Setting

To help all patients increase fertility awareness, we suggest that all primary care providers — including advanced practice nurses, physician assistants, family practice and internal medicine physicians, and obstetrician gynecology specialists — should improve their knowledge of infertility. This is particularly important in communities where patients may not have access to specialized fertility care, and where primary care providers may be the first point of contact for patients seeking information on fertility options. By providing these resources, primary care providers can help to reduce the barriers to accessing fertility care and increase the utilization of these services among all communities, especially those that are underserved and face health disparities. In addition, fertility clinics should provide multilingual pamphlets with easy-to-read information, multilingual short videos, and illustrations on fertility.

Clinics should have diverse providers and staff that mirror their community because this can lead to improved outcomes.[34–41] Diverse perspectives, experiences, and cultural competencies allow inclusive and equitable care for all patients. A meta-analysis of medical and business research concluded that workforce diversity is linked to improved patient outcomes, financial performance, innovation, team communication, and risk assessment, among other factors.[47] Moreover, studies of physicians in other subspecialties suggest that underrepresented minority physicians disproportionately care for patients who identify as minorities, indigent, and uninsured. Specifically, underrepresented minority pediatricians saw nearly 25% more minority patients and more than 10% more Medicaid-insured or uninsured patients than did nonunderrepresented minority pediatricians.[48] Similarly, a survey distributed to 38,133 recertifying family medicine physicians revealed that those who identified as underrepresented minority physicians had larger percentages of underserved patients than did majority physicians.[49,50] Increasing diversity in the physician workforce may reduce disparities in fertility care by promoting a heightened interest in serving patients who share similar backgrounds and experiences.[50]

One solution to increasing diversity within REI is to focus on creating pipelines for physicians from underrepresented groups to enter the field. For example, mentorship programs, scholarships, and outreach programs can all be aimed at encouraging and supporting individuals from diverse backgrounds to pursue careers in reproductive medicine. Additionally, collaborating with community organizations and educational institutions may foster interest among underrepresented groups.

Another strategy is to increase diversity within the leadership and staff of health-care organizations, including reproductive care clinics. To achieve sustainable improvements, we must actively train and promote individuals from diverse backgrounds, create a welcoming and inclusive work environment, provide cultural competency training for staff, promote diversity and inclusion through policies and practices, and encourage open and respectful dialog about diversity and inclusion.

Community

Reducing health disparities in fertility care requires a multifaceted approach. Establishing a sense of community among Black and Hispanic patients may help mitigate disparities by reducing social stigma. This can be achieved through public campaigns and technology-driven resources such as social media platforms and online personalized tools that help connect patients with information and resources. For example, Resolve, a national infertility association, has partnered with ASRM to promote National Infertility Week, traditionally held the last week of April. Providers can collaborate with other national organizations such as Fertility for Colored Girls, The Black Women's Health Imperative, and The Cade Foundation. Additionally, we propose that ART providers conduct targeted, culturally diverse campaigns that focus on destigmatizing infertility within Black and Hispanic communities. Support groups for patients and cultural competency and bias training for health-care providers can help to create a welcoming and inclusive environment for patients from diverse backgrounds. Providing educational activities at schools, colleges, and medical schools helps increase awareness and understanding of fertility care among Black and Hispanic communities and can encourage individuals from these communities to pursue careers in reproductive medicine. By building a sense of community and addressing the unique needs and challenges faced by Black and Hispanic patients, we can help to reduce health disparities in fertility care.

Outcomes

To improve equity in fertility care outcomes, ART providers should work to include more Black and Hispanic patients in data reporting and research studies. We agree with the "universal reporting" of race/ethnicity that was suggested by Wellons and colleagues for all SART data.[30] Consistent reporting of race/ethnicity will allow for more research and a better understanding of the health inequities, followed by focused efforts to eliminate those disparities.

Finally, providers can help achieve equitable ART outcomes by supporting organizations that work to increase access to care through financial support, addressing social determinants of health such as food quality, providing allies that help patients navigate the process of ART in a culturally competent and sensitive way, supporting the emotional stressors that come with ART, providing accurate information, and encouraging patients to actively participate in decision-making regarding their care.

SUMMARY

In conclusion, the disparities in access to fertility care for Black and Hispanic communities are a major public health issue that must be addressed. The solution to reducing these disparities is multifaceted and must involve advocacy, changes in the clinical setting, community outreach, and a focus to improve outcomes. Health-care providers must strive to provide culturally competent care and ensure that their patients have access to accurate and up-to-date information about fertility and infertility treatments. Community outreach programs and public education campaigns may increase fertility knowledge and awareness, reduce the stigma surrounding infertility, and ensure that individuals have access to the resources they need to pursue their reproductive goals.

Finally, advocacy efforts, including policy changes that increase access to care and reduce the cost of treatments, are critical to reducing health disparities in fertility care. By working together, health-care providers, advocates, and communities will allow all individuals to build the families they desire and achieve optimal health and well-being. The elimination of disparities in fertility care is both a moral imperative and a crucial step toward advancing reproductive justice and creating a more equitable and inclusive society.

CLINICS CARE POINTS

- Cultural Competency: Emphasize training for all staff to ensure patients from diverse backgrounds feel understood and respected.
- Multilingual Resources: Provide multilingual fertility information to bridge language barriers.
- Patient Advocacy: Empower underserved patients by encouraging questions and open dialogue.
- Diverse Recruitment: Prioritize recruiting and retaining a workforce that mirrors the diversity of patient populations.
- Quality Improvement: Analyze outcomes for Black and Hispanic patients and address any disparities found.
- Delayed Referrals: Avoid unnecessary delays in fertility evaluations, as timely care can impact treatment success.
- Assuming Reproductive Literacy: Don't presume patients know reproductive health details; provide clear education and explanations.
- Overlooking Racial Concordance: Where feasible, recognize the potential benefits of matching patient-physician racial backgrounds for enhanced patient comfort and understanding.

FUNDING

None.

ACKNOWLEDGMENTS

We thank Deborah Frank, PhD for editorial comments.

DECLARATION OF INTERESTS

All authors has no conflict of interest.

REFERENCES

1. Chandra A, Copen CE, Stephen EH. Infertility and impaired fecundity in the United States, 1982-2010: data from the National Survey of Family Growth. National Heal Statistics Reports 2013;(67):1–18, 1 p following 19.
2. Kelley AS, Qin Y, Marsh EE, et al. Disparities in accessing infertility care in the United States: results from the National Health and Nutrition Examination Survey, 2013–16. Fertil Steril 2019;112(3):562–8.
3. McQueen DB, Schufreider A, Lee SM, et al. Racial disparities in in vitro fertilization outcomes. Fertil Steril 2015;104(2):398–402.e1.
4. Ebeh DN, Jahanfar S. Association between maternal race and the use of assisted reproductive technology in the USA. Sn Compr Clin Medicine 2021;3(5):1106–14.
5. Reindollar RH. Surfing the waves of change in reproductive medicine: past, present and future. A presentation of the 2014 ASRM Strategic Plan. Fertil Steril 2015;103(1):35–8.
6. Medicine TEC of the AS for R. Disparities in access to effective treatment for infertility in the United States: an Ethics Committee opinion. Fertil Steril 2021;116(1): 54–63.

7. Bureau USC. Income in the United States: 2021.; 2022. Accessed February 11, 2023. https://www.census.gov/library/publications/2022/demo/p60-276.html#: ~ : text=Real%20median%20household%20income%20was,and%20Table%20A-1).

8. Koniares KG, Penzias AS, Roosevelt J, et al. The massachusetts infertility insurance mandate: not nearly enough. F S Reports 2022;3(4):305–10.

9. Jain T, Hornstein MD. Disparities in access to infertility services in a state with mandated insurance coverage. Fertil Steril 2005;84(1):221–3.

10. Feinberg EC, Larsen FW, Wah RM, et al. Economics may not explain Hispanic underutilization of assisted reproductive technology services. Fertil Steril 2007; 88(5):1439–41.

11. Quinn M, Fujimoto V. Racial and ethnic disparities in assisted reproductive technology access and outcomes. Fertil Steril 2016;105(5):1119–23.

12. Correia KFB, Kraschel K, Seifer DB. State insurance mandates for in vitro fertilization are not associated with improving racial and ethnic disparities in utilization and treatment outcomes. Am J Obstet Gynecol 2022. https://doi.org/10.1016/j.ajog.2022.10.043.

13. Dieke AC, Zhang Y, Kissin DM, et al. Disparities in assisted reproductive technology utilization by race and ethnicity, United States, 2014: A commentary. J Wom Health 2017;26(6):605–8.

14. Kilfoyle KA, Vitko M, O'Conor R, et al. Health literacy and women's reproductive health: a systematic review. J Wom Health 2016;25(12):1237–55.

15. Literacy I of M (US) C on H. In: Nielsen-Bohlman L, Panzer AM, Kindig DA, editors. Health literacy: a prescription to end confusion. Vol 42. National Academies Press; 2004. https://doi.org/10.5860/choice.42-4059.

16. Meissner C, Schippert C, Versen-Höynck F von. Awareness, knowledge, and perceptions of infertility, fertility assessment, and assisted reproductive technologies in the era of oocyte freezing among female and male university students. J Assist Reprod Genet 2016;33(6):719–29.

17. Pedro J, Brandão T, Schmidt L, et al. What do people know about fertility? A systematic review on fertility awareness and its associated factors. Ups J Med Sci 2018;123(2):1–11.

18. Hoffman JR, Delaney MA, Valdes CT, et al. Disparities in fertility knowledge among women from low and high resource settings presenting for fertility care in two United States metropolitan centers. Fertility Res Pract 2020;6(1):15.

19. Siegel DR, Sheeder J, Polotsky AJ. Racial and ethnic disparities in fertility awareness among reproductive-aged women. Women's Heal Reports 2021;2(1):347–54.

20. Swift BE, Liu KE. The effect of age, ethnicity, and level of education on fertility awareness and duration of infertility. J Obstet Gynaecol Can 2014;36(11):990–6.

21. Insogna IG, Lanes A, Hariton E, et al. Self-reported barriers to accessing infertility care: patient perspectives from urban gynecology clinics. J Assist Reprod Genet 2020;37(12):3007–14.

22. Maher JY, Pal L, Illuzzi JL, et al. Racial and ethnic differences in reproductive knowledge and awareness among women in the United States. F S Reports 2022;3(2):46–54.

23. Wiltshire A, Brayboy LM, Phillips K, et al. Infertility knowledge and treatment beliefs among African American women in an urban community. Contracept Reproductive Medicine 2019;4(1):16.

24. Missmer SA, Seifer DB, Jain T. Cultural factors contributing to health care disparities among patients with infertility in Midwestern United States. Fertil Steril 2011; 95(6):1943–9.

25. Becker G, Castrillo M, Jackson R, et al. Infertility among low-income Latinos. Fertil Steril 2006;85(4):882–7.

26. Chandra A, Martinez GM, Mosher WD, et al. Fertility, family planning, and reproductive health of U.S. women: Data from the 2002 National Survey of Family Growth. Vital Health Stat 2005. https://doi.org/10.1037/e414702008-001.

27. Wellons MF, Lewis CE, Schwartz SM, et al. Racial differences in self-reported infertility and risk factors for infertility in a cohort of black and white women: The CARDIA Women's Study. Fertil Steril 2008;90(5):1640–8.

28. Butts SF. Health disparities of African Americans in reproductive medicine. Fertil Steril 2021;116(2):287–91.

29. Fujimoto VY, Luke B, Brown MB, et al. Racial and ethnic disparities in assisted reproductive technology outcomes in the United States. Fertil Steril 2010;93(2): 382–90.

30. Wellons MF, Fujimoto VY, Baker VL, et al. Race matters: a systematic review of racial/ethnic disparity in Society for Assisted Reproductive Technology reported outcomes. Fertil Steril 2012;98(2):406–9.

31. Ghidei L, Wiltshire A, Raker C, et al. Factors associated with disparate outcomes among Black women undergoing in vitro fertilization. F S Reports 2022;3(2): 14–21.

32. Goodman LR, Balthazar U, Kim J, et al. Trends of socioeconomic disparities in referral patterns for fertility preservation consultation. Hum Reprod 2012;27(7): 2076–81.

33. Kotlyar AM, Simsek B, Seifer DB. Disparities in ART live birth and cumulative live birth outcomes for hispanic and asian women compared to white non-hispanic women. J Clin Medicine 2021;10(12):2615.

34. USA FACTS. Our Changing Population: United States. Published July 1, 2022 Available at: https://usafacts.org/data/topics/people-society/population-and-demographics/our-changing-population/. Accessed August 12, 2023.

35. Cooper-Patrick L, Gallo JJ, Gonzales JJ, et al. Race, gender, and partnership in the patient-physician relationship. JAMA 1999;282(6):583–9.

36. Adams C, Francone N, Chen L, et al. Race/ethnicity and perception of care: does patient–provider concordance matter? Am J Perinatol 2022. https://doi.org/10. 1055/s-0042-1755548.

37. Takeshita J, Wang S, Loren AW, et al. Association of racial/ethnic and gender concordance between patients and physicians with patient experience ratings. JAMA Netw Open 2020;3(11):e2024583.

38. Schoenthaler A, Ravenell J. Understanding the patient experience through the lenses of racial/ethnic and gender patient-physician concordance. JAMA Netw Open 2020;3(11):e2025349.

39. Saha S, Beach MC. Impact of physician race on patient decision-making and ratings of physicians: a randomized experiment using video vignettes. J Gen Intern Med 2020;35(4):1084–91.

40. Meghani SH, Brooks JM, Gipson-Jones T, et al. Patient–provider race-concordance: does it matter in improving minority patients' health outcomes? Ethn Health 2009;14(1):107–30.

41. Otte SV. Improved patient experience and outcomes: is patient–provider concordance the key? J Patient Exp 2022;9. 23743735221103030.

42. Brotherton SE, Etzel SI. Graduate medical education, 2018-2019. JAMA 2019; 322(10):996–1016.

43. Street RL, O'Malley KJ, Cooper LA, et al. Understanding concordance in patient-physician relationships: personal and ethnic dimensions of shared identity. Ann Fam Med 2008;6(3):198–205.

44. Lai JD, Fantus RJ, Cohen AJ, et al. Unmet financial burden of infertility care and the impact of state insurance mandates in the United States: analysis from a popular crowdfunding platform. Fertil Steril 2021;116(4):1119–25.

45. RESOLVE: The National Infertility Association. Insurance Coverage by State. Published June 1, 2023. Accessed August 4, 2023. https://resolve.org/learn/financial-resources-for-family-building/insurance-coverage/insurance-coverage-by-state/.

46. Galic I, Negris O, Warren C, et al. Disparities in access to fertility care: who's in and who's out. F S Reports 2021;2(1):109–17.

47. Gomez LE, Bernet P. Diversity improves performance and outcomes. J Natl Med Assoc 2019;111(4):383–92.

48. Brotherton SE, Stoddard JJ, Tang S, et al. Minority and nonminority pediatricians' care of minority and poor children. Arch Pediatr Adolesc Med 2000;154(9):912–7.

49. Jetty A, Hyppolite J, Eden AR, et al. Underrepresented minority family physicians more likely to care for vulnerable populations. J Am Board Fam Medicine 2022;35(2):223–4.

50. Moy E, Bartman BA. Physician race and care of minority and medically indigent patients. JAMA 1995;273(19):1515–20.

The Role of Artificial Intelligence and Machine Learning in Assisted Reproductive Technologies

Victoria S. Jiang, MD[a,1], Zoran J. Pavlovic, MD[b,1],
Eduardo Hariton, MD, MBA[c],*

KEYWORDS

- Machine learning • Artificial intelligence • IVF • Embryology
- Convolutional neural networks • Support vector machines • Ethics

KEY POINTS

- Understanding the components and important definitions of artificial intelligence.
- AI-based algorithms for the improvement of reproductive medicine.
- Ethical dilemmas and limitations potentially leading to worsening healthcare bias or misdiagnoses.

INTRODUCTION

Artificial intelligence (AI) has become a ubiquitous term, encompassing a broad range of technologies, software, interfaces, and algorithms utilized in big data analytics to forecast outcomes or synthesize information for desired responses. AI mimics human intelligence, using input data to train complex statistical models to generate outputs, much like the human mind processes external sensory perception to form conclusions. In recent years, AI has become a central force driving innovation and entrepreneurship in various fields, including automobile engineering, self-driving vehicles,

Article Type: Literature Review/Systematic Review.
[a] Division of Reproductive Endocrinology & Infertility, Vincent Department of Obstetrics and Gynecology, Massachusetts General Hospital/Harvard Medical School, 55 Fruit Street, Suite 10A, Boston, MA 02116, USA; [b] Department of Obstetrics and Gynecology/Reproductive Endocrinology and Infertility, University of South Florida, Morsani College of Medicine, 2 Tampa General Circle, 6th Floor, Suite 6022, Tampa, FL 33602, USA; [c] Reproductive Science Center of the San Francisco Bay Area, 100 Park Place #200, San Ramon, CA 94583, USA
[1] Both authors contributed equally to this work.
* Corresponding author. Reproductive Science Center of the San Francisco Bay Area, 3300 Webster Street, Suite 404, Oakland, CA 94609.
E-mail address: hariton.md@gmail.com

voice and facial recognition, and healthcare decision-making. Reproductive endocrinology and infertility (REI) is 1such field that has experienced exponential growth in the use of AI for clinical purposes, particularly in overcoming the subjectivity inherent in fertility procedures.[1] While many assume that companies have achieved general AI (GAI), the reality is that we have only scratched the surface of narrow AI (NAI) in medicine, including in REI.[2] In this review, we examine the current and future role of AI and machine learning (ML) in reproductive technologies, exploring exciting solutions to common challenges.

Artificial Intelligence's Medical History

The integration of AI into medicine has a rich history dating back to the 1950s to 60s, with early efforts centered on developing expert systems to aid healthcare professionals in diagnosing and treating diseases. Rule-based algorithms and pre-existing knowledge were the basis for these systems, providing recommendations and decision-making support.[3] In the 1990s, ML and computer vision advancements led to innovative AI applications, including image analysis and computer-aided diagnosis. As computing power and dataset availability grew, deep learning techniques emerged and made substantial improvements in image analysis, natural language processing, and predictive modeling in the 2010s.[3,4] AI has since become an indispensable tool in many areas of medicine, including radiology,[5] dermatology,[6] oncology,[7] and gastroenterology,[8] aimed at improving patient care, reducing costs, and predicting patient outcomes. Despite its promise, the use of AI in clinical practice is still in its infancy, facing several ethical, regulatory, and technical challenges that must be addressed.[9] Nonetheless, AI's potential benefits in medicine are significant, and its use is expected to increase substantially, particularly in assisted reproductive technologies (ART). Early milestones in this development are highlighted in **Fig. 1**.

Artificial Intelligence Definitions and Forms

Understanding basic definitions in the realm of AI is crucial to appreciate where the field of reproductive medicine currently stands. GAI often comes to mind when considering AI (**Table 1**). GAI encompasses the development of machines with human-level intelligence, enabling them to reason, problem-solve, make decisions, understand, and learn like humans. It is an AI system that can perform any intellectual

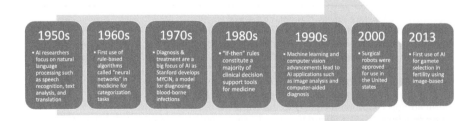

Fig. 1. Timeline of major advances in artificial intelligence over the years. (This figure was adapted from Davenport et al 2019[45] and Chow et al 2021.[46])

Table 1		
Terminology	**Abbreviation**	**Definition**
General Artificial Intelligence (AI)	GAI	• A developed machine algorithm with human-like intelligence such as the ability to reason, problem-solve, make decisions, understand, or learn-like humans capable of performing intellectual tasks. • A wide-form GAI has not yet been achieved in technological development.
Narrow AI	NAI	• A developed machine algorithm that is trained on a dataset to perform a specific task with the limited ability to generalize knowledge learned from training to new unique scenarios. • These systems lack general intelligence but are instead trained on highly specific scenarios or questions and infer output responses from input data used for training. • NAI is the basis of current AI systems used throughout medicine and other fields of interest.
Machine learning	ML	• A subset of AI where an algorithm is trained to learn and make predictions based on training data without explicit programming for a specific task • ML uses statistical techniques to analyze patterns within large datasets to make predictions to address specific scenarios. • Various ML models exist including neural networks (NNs), convolutional neural networks (CNNs), support vectors machines (SVMs), decision trees, random forests (RFs), etc.
Black box AI	Black box AI	• AI algorithms that are opaque in decision-making processes, making it difficult to determine factors that contribute to the given output or decision. • Given challenges in determining contributors to output decision masking, these algorithms may mask biases within the training process or dataset which can lead to flawed decision-making and exacerbate or perpetuate disparities within decision-making particularly in medicine. • By lacking transparency in decision-making, these algorithms make it difficult to assess fairness and accuracy of AI systems.

task a human can, and while theoretic, it remains unachieved in practice. Current AI systems, known as NAI, can only perform specific tasks and are limited in their ability to generalize knowledge to new scenarios like humans.[10]

Presently, the prevailing technology predominantly relies on NAI systems. NAI systems are designed and trained to perform specific tasks, lacking general intelligence, reasoning or understanding abilities like humans.[11] Such systems have a limited range of capabilities as they are trained on specific datasets, excelling at a particular task but struggling with tasks beyond their domain. Examples of NAI include image and speech recognition, as well as language translation systems. Additionally, ML is a subset of AI, enabling computers to learn and make predictions based on data without explicit programming for a specific task. ML algorithms use statistical techniques to analyze patterns in data and make predictions based on those patterns.[12]

In the medical field, NAI and ML are primarily applied through a variety of models, including neural networks (NNs), convolutional neural networks (CNNs), support vector machines (SVMs), decision trees, and random forests (RFs). Among these models, NN, CNN, and SVM are the most used in medical applications. NN is a type of ML model that is inspired by the structure and function of the human brain. It comprises interconnected nodes that work together to process information and make predictions based on weighted connections between nodes that are adjusted during training to learn how to map inputs to outputs.[13] NNs are particularly effective at integrating categorical and continuous variables to generate specific outputs, and are widely used in medical research and diagnosis.

SVMs are a potent class of supervised learning algorithms commonly used for classification and regression analysis. SVMs employ a mathematical construct known as the "hyperplane" to split a dataset into different classes or predict continuous values for regression. The algorithm determines the optimal hyperplane that maximizes the distance between it and the nearest data points of each class, known as support vectors. The SVM adjusts the weights of input features during the training process to find the best hyperplane that separates the data. SVMs can then use this hyperplane to make predictions for new data by determining which side of the hyperplane the data fall on.[12] SVMs are commonly employed in medical research to predict treatment outcomes and diagnose diseases, such as predicting breast cancer risk[14] and diagnosing heart diseases.[15]

CNNs are the game-changers of image and video processing in the world of deep learning.[16] With a profound ability to recognize and classify objects, voices, and even faces, their impact cannot be overstated. In embryology, where the smallest morphologic changes may hold significant importance, CNNs are indispensable for image processing in ART. They serve as the backbone of many AI algorithms within the fertility industry, precisely evaluating gametes and embryos' competency, aiding in selection, and predicting implantation potential.[16] The algorithm architecture, complexity and suitability of NNs and CNNs vary significantly from SVMs. While SVMs work well with smaller datasets, NNs and CNNs have a multi-layered architecture that is best suited for more extensive, non-linear datasets.

The advent of algorithms, imaging systems, software, and workflow initiatives has ushered in a new era of clinical decision-making, transforming ART in unprecedented ways. With these AI-driven tools, clinicians can optimize gonadotropin starting doses, analyze the competency and quality of embryos or oocytes, and even predict individualized in vitro fertilization (IVF) outcomes with greater precision than ever before. However, as rapid innovations continue to shape the field of REI, it is essential to take stock of the current state of the art, anticipate future developments, and identify the ethical, practical, and technical challenges that must be overcome to improve patient safety, care, and outcomes. This review delves deeper into these applications, shedding light on their potential to revolutionize the fertility industry.[16]

ARTIFICIAL INTELLIGENCE INNOVATIONS & APPLICATIONS

The integration of AI into ART has been nothing short of revolutionary, opening a world of new possibilities for clinical medicine. From patient consultation to embryo transfer, AI-powered solutions have transformed every aspect of ART, particularly in the realm of IVF. With cutting-edge research now unlocking its full potential, AI promises to revolutionize IVF stimulation cycles in ways we could scarcely have imagined before. This section delves into the numerous, exciting applications of AI within the IVF stimulation cycle, exploring the potential of this game-changing technology.

In Vitro Fertilization Stimulation

In the past half-decade, the field of ART has witnessed an explosion of innovative AI platforms designed to optimize every aspect of the IVF process. One crucial step in this process is selecting the appropriate starting gonadotropin dosage and dose adjustments, which can significantly improve patient outcomes and reduce overall costs. However, the subjective nature of these decisions often leads to wide variations in clinical practice. To address this challenge, Fanton and colleagues[17] developed an interpretable ML model that leveraged data from over 18,500 IVF cycles to create dose-responsive models using the k-nearest neighbors (k-NN) model.[17] Both their dose-responsive and flat-responsive models were shown to be effective in selecting lower doses of starting follicle stimulating hormone (FSH) and total FSH dosing, leading to more MII oocytes, 2 pronuclei (PN) embryos, and useable blastocysts, using a lower dose, which would result in lower average cost per patient.

In terms of how to manage patient visits, Letterie and colleagues[18] developed a decision support system AI framework to assess 4 major decision points within the IVF cycle, such as when to continue or stop stimulation, trigger or cancel treatment, the number of days for follow-up, and subsequent need for dose adjustment.[18] In a direct comparison with 12 clinicians, the algorithm achieved high accuracies of 0.92 for continue or stop treatment, 0.96 for trigger/cancel/proceed to retrieval, 0.82 for medication dose adjustment, and 0.87 for the number of days to follow-up.[18] This study suggests that AI can help predict the right intervals of time between appointments, allowing for streamlining of patient care. Future models could be optimized not only to replicate physician behavior, but to minimize visits without compromising outcomes or safety, potentially leading to cost savings and improvements in patient experience.

Various algorithms have been developed to optimize trigger timing in ART which may lead to significant improvements in clinical outcomes. In a seminal study, Hariton and colleagues[19] demonstrated that when compared to the physicians' decision, a bagged decision tree model trained to choose trigger timing could increase the number of 2PNs and useable blastocysts by approximately 3 and 1.5, respectively. When compared to the physician's decisions, the model's recommendations resulted in an improvement of 1.4 more 2PNs and 0.6 more useable blastocysts per stimulation when applied to 7866 patients. Another study by Fanton and colleagues[20] used a linear regression ML model to assess the effect of early and late trigger timing on 30,278 patients. After propensity scoring, this study revealed that early and late triggers resulted in fewer MII oocytes, 2PNs, and useable blastocysts than optimal triggers, emphasizing the role AI-aided decision-making may play in improving ART outcomes.

Optimizing workflow and level-loading for individual stimulation management is critical as clinical volumes continue to rise globally. Level-loading is a term borrowed from the manufacturing industry where lean operations are prioritized thereby reducing waste. The premise lies in the notion that spreading out the production, assembly and shipping of a product evenly over the course of a week, month, quarter, or all of the aforementioned would ultimately be more efficient and reduce waste than a chaotic nearing-a-deadline approach. In the field of fertility this would be comparable to spreading patient monitoring and retrievals out more evenly over a month rather than having idle patient care days interspersed between overwhelming clinic schedules. Letterie and colleagues[21] introduced an innovative approach to address this issue, utilizing patient clinical parameters to identify the optimal day for monitoring, trigger date, and ranges for 3 oocyte retrieval dates for level-loading while estimating the number of retrieved oocytes. What's unique about this model is that it uses the number of oocytes retrieved to determine the earliest and latest day of trigger, minimizing the variance of 0 to 3 oocytes. This bird's eye view application of ML tackles the 3 critical nodal points of decision-making in workflow optimization, potentially reducing time spent monitoring and level-loading the embryology workflow while still maintaining clinical outcomes.

Follicular Monitoring

Ultrasound monitoring of ovarian follicular growth is a crucial but time-consuming component of ART or IVF, affecting patients and clinics' efficiency, costs per cycle, disruption of patients' professional work schedules, and general discomfort from invasive testing procedures such as laboratory draws and transvaginal ultrasound monitoring. Previous attempts at automating the process involved segmenting 2-dimensional ultrasound images to identify follicular contours using computer tracking devices. Recently, some clinics are shifting to 3-dimensional ultrasonographic imaging, with segmentation-based AI algorithms able to measure follicular size and optimize trigger timing. These algorithms have been shown to significantly reduce the time needed per follicular ultrasound in comparison to manual monitoring. Moreover, deep learning applications have shown promising results in accurately tracking follicle size with correlations of up to 98% for different follicle sizes.[22–25] By reducing the resources spent on monitoring, automated follicular monitoring can improve efficiency and reduce costs for both patients and clinics, while maintaining clinical outcomes. Furthermore, standardizing the follicle measurement inputs for stimulation models can further reduce noise and improve the effectiveness of AI tools.

Embryo Selection

Image analysis using ML algorithms such as CNNs has revolutionized how a developing zygote is evaluated within the embryology laboratory. Current embryo selection methods consist of employing various embryo grading systems to indicate embryo quality, with higher quality embryos receiving a priority for transfer (DOI 10.1097/00001703-199906000-00013 and 10.1007/s43032-020-00389-y). Additionally, preimplantation genetic testing (PGT) can be employed to select for euploid embryos which have a higher live birth rate when compared to untested embryos in various patient populations (https://doi.org/10.1016/j.rbmo.2021.09.011). When it comes to embryo grading, embryologists are relied upon to make subjective judgements, and certain imaging advancements have been utilized to try and diminish intra-observer and inter-observer variation (doi:10.1016/j.rbmo.2021.08.008). AI has the potential to further improve this process. The visual aspects of embryo development in both still and video forms are ripe for the exponential image processing capabilities of CNNs, affording new advances in embryo grading, predicting implantation potential, and clinical decision-making at critical time points like when to freeze, discard, or biopsy. Embryo evaluation initially aimed at automatic blastocyst grading using time-lapse imaging. CNN and recurrent neural networks (RNNs) evaluating video-based data have been described with near human accuracy for blastocyst grading.[26] Implantation potential, defined as the likelihood of clinical pregnancy following transfer of a selected blastocyst, was a natural extension of this technology. Bormann and colleagues[27] utilized CNNs to evaluate single-timepoint embryo images and showed that among 97 clinical patient cohorts of 742 embryos; the CNN was able to accurately select the highest quality embryo with a 90% accuracy, consistently outperforming 15 trained embryologists from 5 different centers. In 1of the largest studies of its kind, VerMilyea et al[28] describe Life Whisperer AI, a CNN-based algorithm trained on over 8800 embryos from 11 different IVF centers across 3 countries can select viable embryos with a sensitivity of 70.1%, with an overall weighted accuracy of more than 63%, showing the generalizability of algorithms to a wide range of data. With many groups continuing to develop and publish algorithms with increasing accuracy, we are reaching a renaissance of technological development that will change the scope of embryo selection to be more efficient, lowering cost and time needed within the laboratory. Optimizing embryo selection, particularly euploid embryo selection, may decrease costs and potentially lead to few cycles per patient to achieve pregnancy, allowing clinics to extend care to more patients.

Inter-observer subjectivity is a major challenge of any visual-based field, with decision-making impacting subsequent outcomes and pregnancy rates. While top quality and non-viable embryos can be reliably selected between embryologists,[29,30] blastocysts with borderline appearance can have significant inter-observer variability, with 1 study showing agreement among 18 embryologist as low at 52.7%.[29] These borderline blastocysts can be the most challenging to evaluate and grade, where high inter-observer variability from personal subjectivity can lead to detrimental consequences for patients and clinics alike. If a borderline blastocyst is graded as not of quality to cryopreserve or transfer, this may be eliminating a viable blastocyst capable of producing a successful pregnancy, lowering the number of embryos per cycle. In the most extreme cases, if only borderline blastocysts are made in this context, this may eliminate all embryos available for transfer, biopsy, or cryopreservation, which is particularly detrimental in cases of limited ovarian reserve or when electing for any type of PGT. Alternatively, electing to cryopreserve or transfer borderline blastocysts that some would deem low quality may also be harmful. From the patient perspective, if cryopreserved with plans for future PGT or transfer, these borderline blastocysts may be creating a sense of false hope, leading to loss of time in either performing another cycle or in costly repetitive, unsuccessful transfer cycles. In older patients or patients with limited ovarian reserve, this loss of time can mean the difference between using autologous oocytes for future cycles or necessitating donor oocyte utilization, increasing psychological, emotional, and financial burden among patients. Furthermore, these embryos will likely not be initially prioritized for transfer given lower initial grade. If a patient has completed family building, leftover embryos can lead to challenges in embryo disposition decisions, resulting in either eternal financial costs of yearly storage fees or the need for thaw/discard/donation. From a clinic perspective, biopsying and/or cryopreserving these embryos which are likely futile lead to increased work-load and need for cryopreservation space within laboratiries, increasing the cost per clinic while simultaneously physically taxing an already busy embryology laboratory. Gamete and embryo storage has been a growing challenge for clinics, as the need for long-term storage space is commonly constrained by physical clinic space. Further, offsite storage has been a solution in some situations, risking gametes and embryos to transportation and logistical risks, not to mention the continual organizational demands of tracking and maintaining accurate storage logs. For these reasons, borderline blastocysts can be most challenging to disposition or manage, and decreasing subjectivity among embryologists is an essential goal in increasing the efficiency of the ART process and the IVF laboratory.

Decreasing this subjectivity and improving selection methods through AI-assistance to optimize implantation will improve both clinical outcomes and efficiency within the laboratory. AI helps eliminate a degree of subjectivity in embryo selection, commonly outperforming embryologists in embryo selection for implantation potential or euploidy. When directly compared to embryologists in 200 sets of day 5 euploid embryo images, AI algorithms have lesser variability in selections, and can select successfully implanted embryos in 73.6% of cases, significantly higher than the 65.5%

selected on visual assessment by embryologist alone.[31] Most strikingly, however, this study showed that AI-aided decision-making improved all embryologist selections on average by 11.1%,[31] showing the power of AI assistance alongside the embryologist, rather than instead of the embryologist.

Implantation potential, while valuable in embryo selection, cannot be fully evaluated in isolation from genetic aneuploidy. With implantation potential as an important stepping stone for algorithm development, the next step naturally would be evaluating the use of AI for non-invasive ploidy prediction, such euploid/aneuploid classification. Notably, utilizing AI for embryo selection has the potential to expand options for non-invasive screening, an important tool, especially in geographies where there is limited access to PGT-A due to cost or technical limitations. With the increasing costs of IVF worldwide in a growing add-on market, non-invasive genetic screening with AI can potentially serve as a cheaper, more efficient, resource-friendly option that can provide same-day results for embryo selection prior to transfer. In a small cohort of around 400 patients, Yuan and colleagues[32] reported a logistic regression-based ML model that was able to predict euploidy with an area under the curve of 0.879. This model, however, was unable to predict live birth after frozen embryo transfer. In the largest studies to date tackling this issue, Barnes and colleagues[33] describe their model, STORK-A, which combines deep learning and ML methods such as extreme gradient boost decision tree, k-NN, SVM, and RFs to assess embryo morphology, morphokinetics, and associate cycle information such as maternal age to predict euploidy, single aneuploidy, and complex aneuploidy. This model was trained and validated from over 10,000 embryos from both the United States and Spain and predicted aneuploidy vs euploidy with an accuracy of 69.3%.[33] Two additional models were created to assess complex aneuploidy versus euploidy versus single aneuploidy and complex aneuploidy versus euploidy with accuracies of 74.0% and 77.6%, respectively.[33] With average performance accuracy between 60% and 75% in most reported algorithms, dynamic weighted voting, such as the use of voting ensembles, serves as a potential method for improving accuracy of pre-existing models. In a novel application, Jiang and colleagues[34] showed that using voting ensembles to combine CNN-based image analysis with SVM and NN-based analysis of cycle characteristics can increase the performance accuracy by over 10%. Combining different ML algorithms allows for a larger variety of variable analysis from morphology alone, serving as a potential non-invasive method to aid in karyotype screening and embryo selection. While current algorithms do not yet have the accuracy to reliably predict aneuploidy as a stand-alone test, the promise of these technologies is wide-reaching as a potential adjunct to morphology-only selection. Furthermore, combining these technologies with other emerging ones, such as spent media analysis and morphokinetics, may improve the performance beyond what a single 1 can do alone.

Quality Assurance Within Embryology

AI is being increasingly utilized in the field of quality assurance (QA) within embryology laboratories, with a focus on evaluating embryo morphology using visual NNs such as CNNs and RNNs. These QA models use key performance indicators (KPIs) to monitor and evaluate embryologists, providers, and the embryo culture system, allowing for the identification of areas for improvement that may impact clinical outcomes. By objectively assessing embryo morphology, AI algorithms can predict outcomes such as blastocyst formation and implantation potential, enabling direct comparisons with real-time outcomes and providing more rapid assessment and corrections within the clinic or culture system.

One novel application of AI for QA was described by Bormann and colleagues[35] in 2021, where a CNN was trained to predict the likelihood of blastocyst development and used to evaluate the impact of different media lots and embryologists performing intracytoplasmic sperm injection (ICSI) on blastocyst formation rates. By comparing predicted and actual blastocyst formation rates, areas for QA assessment were identified. AI can also be used to evaluate medical providers' and embryologists' performance in clinical procedures, such as embryo transfer, embryo vitrification, and trophectoderm biopsy.[36] Regular evaluations using AI can streamline the QA process and reduce delays in identifying areas for improvement, ultimately improving clinical outcomes.

Gamete and Embryo Witnessing

Accurate identification and handling of patient gametes and embryos is critical in the embryology laboratory to ensure patient safety and avoid malpractice litigation. While the current standard of care for embryo identification is double witnessing by 2 embryology staff members, advancements in technology have allowed for additional safeguards such as radio frequency identification and embryo tagging. However, recent advancements in AI have opened up new possibilities for accurate and efficient embryo identification.

Using a combination of a CNN trained to identify implantation potential and another CNN trained in genetic identification, day 3 cleavage stage and day 5 blastocyst embryos were identified with 100% accuracy.[37] This remarkable accuracy, if integrated into a laboratory's imaging system, can provide an important safety measure for embryologists, physicians, and patients to ensure accurate identification of embryos. With AI serving as an additional "eye" for witnessing, it can serve as the first to identify the contents within the dish, rather than the dish itself. Thus, the integration of AI into the embryology laboratory has the potential to greatly enhance patient safety and reduce the risk of embryo mix-ups or swaps.

CAN ARTIFICIAL INTELLIGENCE BE INTELLIGENT AND ETHICAL?

As with any major scientific breakthrough, it is crucial to critically consider biases and ethical concerns before widespread adoption, particularly when the technology in question has a direct impact on healthcare and personal medical outcomes (**Table 2**). AI, often touted as an objective decision-making tool, is not exempt from ethical challenges. Developing an AI system requires vast amounts of data, raising concerns about data ownership, privacy, and compliance with Health Insurance Portability and Accountability Act regulations, as well as potential misuse by large data mining companies. It is essential to validate AI software thoroughly, particularly given the inherent bias and variability present in AI models, before using it for clinical decision-making or assistance. A "collapse of an algorithm" is a real concern for new systems trained on poorly optimized datasets. Furthermore, it is unclear whether AI-based technology will serve as a valuable aid for clinicians, embryologists, and patients or whether it will be recklessly pushed as a replacement for human expertise.

It is crucial to acknowledge that despite the perception of objectivity, AI technology is not immune to bias. The AI model is constrained by the proficiency of its creators and the training dataset selected. Human biases are introduced when selecting variables for the AI model, which can potentially exclude significant variables and add confounding variables to the system. Furthermore, the quality of imaging inputs can be restricted by the imaging platform, image annotations, or resolution. To create an adequate training set, clinical outcomes must be meticulously documented, which

Table 2
Common types of biases within artificial intelligence

Bias Category	Specific Bias	Definition
AI Systems Bias	Collapse of Algorithm	Failure to produce meaningful or diverse results, often giving the same or very similar outputs regardless of the variety in the input data.
	Algorithmic Design	Bias that can be introduced by the choices made in algorithm design or in the loss functions and metrics used for evaluation.
	Feedback Loop	When predictions made by the model are fed back into the system, reinforcing the model's beliefs even if those beliefs are not true.
	Anchoring	A cognitive bias where decisions are unduly influenced by initial information, even when subsequent information is presented, thereby preventing improvements in a model.
Data Bias	Sampling	Occurs when the data gathered for analysis are not representative of the population intended to be analyzed.
	Historical	When past prejudices and discriminations are reflected in the data. For instance, if a hiring tool is trained on historical data from a company that have a history of gender bias, the model may replicate that bias.
	Selection	Results from the non-random selection of data that can misrepresent information about a population.
Pre-processing and Algorithmic Bias	Label	Occurs when the labels used in supervised learning are subjective or contain errors.
	Measurement	Errors that result from the data collection process, such as faulty equipment or subjective human measurements.
	Aggregation	When granular data are oversimplified by grouping into broader categories. Oversimplification of data can decrease variance in algorithms and therefore be less useful in complex scenarios.
	Confirmation	When models are designed in a way that they confirm pre-existing beliefs, prejudices, or hypotheses of the researchers.
Post-processing and Deployment Bias	Exclusion	When a model systematically excludes particular groups, often due to them being underrepresented in the training data.
	Extrapolation	When a model makes predictions about situations that are outside the range of the data it was trained on.
Demographic Bias	Societal and Cultural	Prejudices and stereotypes embedded in society can be reflected in AI and ML models, especially if they are trained on data generated by human biases or subjectivity.
	Representation	When certain categories or classes in the data are overrepresented or underrepresented.

may be challenging for certain scenarios, such as untransferred cryopreserved blastocysts, resulting in limited available data for subjective morphology-selected blastocysts. Additionally, the high financial burden of IVF limits access, leading to a known socioeconomic and racial skew among patients in the United States and globally.[38]

It is imperative to recognize that bias can infiltrate every stage of development in AI programs and reflect systemic discrimination. This issue often goes unaddressed, as it contradicts the prevailing belief that technology, including AI, is an impartial and equitable system that does not replicate the flaws of society. One of the initial areas where AI-based algorithms can fall short is inbuilt bias or variance in the training data. AI bias and variance refer to the accuracy and stability of the algorithm, and the objective is to balance out bias and variance as effectively as possible. A biased algorithm oversimplifies the connection between input and output data, leading to underfitting and unsuitability to handle intricate datasets with numerous and subtle relationships between data points. Variance denotes an algorithm's sensitivity to small changes, or "noise," in the training data, causing overfitting, increased specialization at the expense of generalizability, and inaccurate prediction of outcomes from new, unseen input data. An ideal algorithm seeks an appropriate level of complexity and flexibility that neither oversimplifies relationships nor ignores legitimate patterns in the data.[39] The validation of a new dataset and the risk of erratic predictions or algorithm collapse remain significant challenges in current literature. Data privacy and sharing concerns make external validation of any AI algorithm challenging, and caution must be exercised when evaluating any new AI system.

To ensure the safe and ethical deployment of NAI in healthcare, it is crucial for both developers and healthcare professionals to be aware of the impact of bias and variance within algorithms. Biases can be introduced at various stages of algorithm development, and can perpetuate socioeconomic, demographic, and racial inequalities in healthcare delivery.[40] Thus, it is essential for clinicians to ensure that the algorithms used in their practice are as unbiased as possible to prevent the exacerbation of existing healthcare inequalities. Algorithmic collapse, which can occur due to underfitting/overfitting of data or a poor training dataset, is another significant concern for the development of NAI systems. It is essential to create a training dataset that accurately reflects the clinical scenario and that is diverse enough to be generalizable to various patient populations. The lack of diversity in training data can lead to biased algorithms that fail to consider the nuances of patient care and can ultimately impact patient outcomes. Therefore, it is critical to ensure that NAI algorithms are developed with appropriate care and rigor to ensure that they meet ethical standards and promote patient-centered care.

NAI/ML algorithms are highly susceptible to biases due to the training data they receive. Biases can arise from sampling, historical, label, and algorithmic factors. Sampling bias occurs when the training data are not representative of the population they are meant to serve, which can lead to models that fail to accurately reflect the experiences and needs of certain groups. Historical bias results when algorithms are trained on data reflecting patterns of discrimination and inequality, causing models to perform poorly when applied to more diverse patient populations. Label bias occurs when the labels used to train an AI system are biased or discriminatory. For example, a model trained on data that incorrectly attribute symptoms to gender can perpetuate discrimination. Finally, algorithmic bias occurs when biased data are used to train an AI system, leading to inaccurate predictions.[38] In ART, a polygenic risk scoring system trained on a predominantly white population could fail to accurately predict risk in African American patients. As such, it is essential to scrutinize the training data and minimize biases to ensure optimal algorithm performance.

The United Kingdom's use of live facial recognition software to screen for criminal or concerning individuals showed a staggering 81% failure rate, with alarming levels of biased outcomes against minority groups.[41] Similarly, in reproductive medicine, embryo-selection algorithms trained on data from clinic-specific incubators can lead to suboptimal results and a need for more patient-specific algorithms.[42] To combat such biases, it is essential to ensure that AI datasets are representative, diverse, and free from discrimination. This requires incorporating fairness and accountability considerations into the design and development of AI systems, conducting regular audits of the data and algorithms, and using data from a variety of sources to mitigate inherent biases. Failure to do so will perpetuate discriminatory practices, further marginalize vulnerable populations, and undermine the credibility of AI technology in healthcare and other fields.

Black box AI refers to algorithms that are opaque in their decision-making processes, making it difficult to determine the factors that contribute to a given output. In the context of reproductive medicine and IVF, the use of black box AI raises concerns about the potential for bias to go undetected and exacerbate existing healthcare disparities. Without transparency into the underlying algorithms and data sources, it may be difficult to assess the accuracy and fairness of AI systems. Moreover, there is a risk of over-reliance on AI systems, with clinicians and patients failing to question the outputs or seek additional information. This may lead to unintended consequences and harm, such as perpetuating stereotypes, ignoring relevant factors, or inadvertently creating new biases. To address these risks, there is a need for increased transparency and accountability in the development and use of AI systems in reproductive medicine, with clear communication of the potential benefits and limitations, as well as regular auditing and monitoring to detect and correct any biases that arise.

The importance of representative and diverse training data for NAI cannot be overstated. It is vital that these algorithms are trained correctly within intended patient populations to avoid perpetuating biases and discriminatory practices. However, this data requirement brings up a significant concern regarding the ownership and use of patient data.[43] As more patient information is collected, the importance of storing, utilizing, and implementing data appropriately cannot be overlooked. Patients have a right to know how their data are being used and if they are being utilized to produce algorithms that are not discriminatory. In the reproductive medicine space, commercial interests are increasingly entering healthcare, and patient data are becoming a valuable commodity. As such, protecting patient privacy and agency and maintaining data anonymity is of utmost importance. Breach of patient autonomy and anonymity can lead to erosion of patient trust, which has significant implications for patient care. It is crucial that safeguards are developed at national and international levels to ensure appropriate data usage by private entities, academic and research institutions, governments, and most importantly, patient end-users.[44]

THE FUTURE OF ARTIFICIAL INTELLIGENCE-BASED SYSTEMS

With continuously improving performance accuracy and ever-expanding applications, AI can serve as an important tool for a variety of indications within the fertility field. Starting with predictive analytics and stimulation tools, AI can assist providers for more data-driven, unbiased, and streamlined decision-making that can improve patient care. If non-fellowship trained providers participate in ART patient care, AI could serve as a layer of safety to help support them. After retrieval, AI could support embryologists in streamlining laboratory functions and helping select the best embryos for transfers, ideally without needing expensive, invasive procedures such as a trophectoderm biopsy. In conjunction, these technologies can help streamline care by optimizing patient flow, level-loading laboratory volumes, and monitoring clinical and laboratory KPIs to ensure optimal performance and identify deviations early.

While the progress made in this field in the last few years has been very promising, it is important to acknowledge that the field remains in its infancy. The studies discussed previously are excellent proofs of concept that merit continuous investment of time and resources into this area. Nonetheless, they should not be confused with technology capable of immediate integration or widespread adoption. Each algorithm should be systematically tested prospectively to ensure it performs as expected and leads to the accurate, precise, and reproducible outcomes.

Lastly, as we move into a world where computers are an integral part of our decision making, we will have to think deeply about how we continue to train providers and how do we ensure that we are still able to care for patients that do not follow traditional patterns. Furthermore, as automation becomes a reality, we will need to refocus the efforts of our existing and growing workforce to serve patients in different ways such as supervisory or managerial roles, further extending access of care with a limited staff. While the era of AI will bring a lot of positives to our field, it will not come without challenges that we, as a community, will need to manage. Interest groups such as the AI interest group for the American Society of Reproductive Medicine and organizations such as the newly minted AI Fertility Society are appropriate venues for engaging in these discussions which will inevitably shape the future of our field.

SUMMARY

In conclusion, AI and ML have the potential to revolutionize the field of reproductive medicine, providing doctors with powerful tools to enhance patient care, improve outcomes, and increase the standard of care. As this technology continues to evolve, it is essential that we remain vigilant in ensuring that it is well-validated and used ethically. While there is still much to be learned about the use of AI and ML in reproductive medicine, the possibilities are truly exciting, offering a promising positive impact on the lives of patients and families in the years to come. By embracing this new technology responsibly, we can work toward a future in which reproductive medicine is more accessible and effective than ever before.

CLINICS CARE POINTS

- Leveraging AI for Reproductive Medicine: AI presents opportunities to enhance reproductive medicine through improved oocyte and embryo grading, as well as more accurate follicular measurement.

- Individualized Patient Care: AI can aid clinicians in providing individualized care, benefiting both clinicians and patients in achieving the best possible outcomes.

- Bias and Healthcare Inequities: Despite the potential strengths of AI, it is crucial to recognize that algorithms are not immune to bias and may perpetuate socioeconomic and demographic biases present in current healthcare systems

---

CONFLICT OF INTEREST

None.

FUNDING STATEMENT

This study received no financial support.

REFERENCES

1. Riegler MA, Stensen MH, Witczak O, et al. Artificial intelligence in the fertility clinic: status, pitfalls and possibilities. Hum Reprod 2021;36:2429–42.
2. Shortliffe EH. Artificial Intelligence in Medicine: Weighing the Accomplishments, Hype, and Promise. Yearb Med Inform 2019;28:257–62.
3. Kaul V, Enslin S, Gross SA. History of artificial intelligence in medicine. Gastrointest Endosc 2020;92:807–12.
4. Iqbal JD, Vinay R. Are we ready for Artificial Intelligence in Medicine? Swiss Med Wkly 2022;152:w30179.
5. Kelly BS, Judge C, Bollard SM, et al. Radiology artificial intelligence: a systematic review and evaluation of methods (RAISE). Eur Radiol 2022;32:7998–8007.
6. Hogarty DT, Su JC, Phan K, et al. Artificial Intelligence in Dermatology—Where We Are and the Way to the Future: A Review. Am J Clin Dermatol 2020;21:41–7.
7. Kann BH, Hosny A, Aerts HJWL. Artificial intelligence for clinical oncology. Cancer Cell 2021;39:916–27.
8. Kröner PT, Engels MM, Glicksberg BS, et al. Artificial intelligence in gastroenterology: A state-of-the-art review. World J Gastroenterol 2021;27:6794–824.
9. LeonidN Yasnitsky. Artificial Intelligence and Medicine: History, Current State, and Forecasts for the Future. Curr Hypertens Rev 2021;16:210–5.
10. Bohannon J. Fears of an AI pioneer. Science 2015;349:252.
11. Hamet P, Tremblay J. Artificial intelligence in medicine. Metabolism 2017;69: S36–40.
12. Deo RC. Machine Learning in Medicine. Circulation 2015;132:1920–30.
13. Kriegeskorte N, Golan T. Neural network models and deep learning. Curr Biol 2019;29:R231–6.
14. Ibrahim A, Gamble P, Jaroensri R, et al. Artificial intelligence in digital breast pathology: Techniques and applications. Breast 2020;49:267–73.
15. Dash M, Londhe ND, Ghosh S, et al. Swarm intelligence based clustering technique for automated lesion detection and diagnosis of psoriasis. Comput Biol Chem 2020;86:107247.
16. Coleman S, Kerr D, Zhang Y. Image Sensing and Processing with Convolutional Neural Networks. Sensors 2022;22:3612.
17. Fanton M, Nutting V, Rothman A, et al. An interpretable machine learning model for individualized gonadotrophin starting dose selection during ovarian stimulation. Reprod Biomed Online 2022;45:1152–9.
18. Letterie G, Mac Donald A. Artificial intelligence in in vitro fertilization: a computer decision support system for day-to-day management of ovarian stimulation during in vitro fertilization. Fertil Steril 2020;114:1026–31.
19. Hariton E, Chi EA, Chi G, et al. A machine learning algorithm can optimize the day of trigger to improve in vitro fertilization outcomes. Fertil Steril 2021;116:1227–35.
20. Fanton M, Nutting V, Solano F, et al. An interpretable machine learning model for predicting the optimal day of trigger during ovarian stimulation. Fertil Steril 2022; 118:101–8.
21. Letterie G, MacDonald A, Shi Z. An artificial intelligence platform to optimize workflow during ovarian stimulation and IVF: process improvement and outcome-based predictions. Reprod Biomed Online 2022;44:254–60.

22. Liang X, Liang J, Zeng F, et al. Evaluation of oocyte maturity using artificial intelligence quantification of follicle volume biomarker by three-dimensional ultrasound. Reprod Biomed Online 2022;45:1197–206.

23. Mathur P, Kakwani K, Diplav, et al. Deep Learning based Quantification of Ovary and Follicles using 3D Transvaginal Ultrasound in Assisted Reproduction. In: 42nd annu int conf IEEE eng med biol soc EMBC. Montreal, QC, Canada: IEEE; 2020. p. 2109–12. Available at: https://ieeexplore.ieee.org/document/9176703/.

24. Noor N, Vignarajan C, Malhotra N, et al. Three-dimensional automated volume calculation (sonography-based automated volume count) versus two-dimensional manual ultrasonography for follicular tracking and oocyte retrieval in women undergoing in vitro fertilization-embryo transfer: a randomized controlled trial. J Hum Reprod Sci 2020;13:296.

25. Srivastava D, Gupta S, Kudavelly S, et al. Unsupervised Deep Learning based Longitudinal Follicular Growth Tracking during IVF Cycle using 3D Transvaginal Ultrasound in Assisted Reproduction. In: 43rd annu int conf IEEE eng med biol soc EMBC [internet]. Mexico: IEEE; 2021. p. 3209–12. Available at: https://ieeexplore.ieee.org/document/9630495/.

26. Kragh MF, Rimestad J, Berntsen J, et al. Automatic grading of human blastocysts from time-lapse imaging. Comput Biol Med 2019;115:103494.

27. Bormann CL, Kanakasabapathy MK, Thirumalaraju P, et al. Performance of a deep learning based neural network in the selection of human blastocysts for implantation. Elife 2020;9:e55301.

28. VerMilyea M, Hall JMM, Diakiw SM, et al. Development of an artificial intelligence-based assessment model for prediction of embryo viability using static images captured by optical light microscopy during IVF. Hum Reprod 2020;35:770–84.

29. Hammond ER, Foong AKM, Rosli N, et al. Should we freeze it? Agreement on fate of borderline blastocysts is poor and does not improve with a modified blastocyst grading system. Hum Reprod 2020;35:1045–53.

30. Fordham DE, Rosentraub D, Polsky AL, et al. Embryologist agreement when assessing blastocyst implantation probability: is data-driven prediction the solution to embryo assessment subjectivity? Hum Reprod 2022;37:2275–90.

31. Fitz VW, Kanakasabapathy MK, Thirumalaraju P, et al. Should there be an "AI" in TEAM? Embryologists selection of high implantation potential embryos improves with the aid of an artificial intelligence algorithm. J Assist Reprod Genet 2021;38:2663–70.

32. Yuan Z, Yuan M, Song X, et al. Development of an artificial intelligence based model for predicting the euploidy of blastocysts in PGT-A treatments. Sci Rep 2023;13:2322.

33. Barnes J, Brendel M, Gao VR, et al. A non-invasive artificial intelligence approach for the prediction of human blastocyst ploidy: a retrospective model development and validation study. Lancet Digit Health 2023;5:e28–40.

34. Jiang VS, Kandula H, Thirumalaraju P, et al. The use of voting ensembles to improve the accuracy of deep neural networks as a non-invasive method to predict embryo ploidy status. J Assist Reprod Genet 2023;40:301–8.

35. Bormann CL, Curchoe CL, Thirumalaraju P, et al. Deep learning early warning system for embryo culture conditions and embryologist performance in the ART laboratory. J Assist Reprod Genet 2021;38:1641–6.

36. Cherouveim P, Jiang VS, Kanakasabapathy MK, et al. Quality assurance (QA) for monitoring the performance of assisted reproductive technology (ART) staff using artificial intelligence (AI). J Assist Reprod Genet 2023;40:241–9.

37. Hammer KC, Jiang VS, Kanakasabapathy MK, et al. Using artificial intelligence to avoid human error in identifying embryos: a retrospective cohort study. J Assist Reprod Genet 2022;39:2343–8.

38. Fletcher RR, Nakeshimana A, Olubeko O. Addressing Fairness, Bias, and Appropriate Use of Artificial Intelligence and Machine Learning in Global Health. Front Artif Intell 2021;3:561802.

39. Geis JR, Brady AP, Wu CC, et al. Ethics of Artificial Intelligence in Radiology: Summary of the Joint European and North American Multisociety Statement. Radiology 2019;293:436–40.

40. Beam AL, Kohane IS. Big Data and Machine Learning in Health Care. JAMA 2018;319:1317.

41. Fussey P, Murray D. Independent report on the London metropolitan police service's trial of live facial recognition technology [internet]. University of Essex; 2019. Available at: https://repository.essex.ac.uk/24946/1/London-Met-Police-Trial-of-Facial-Recognition-Tech-Report-2.pdf.

42. Barrie A, Homburg R, McDowell G, et al. Examining the efficacy of six published time-lapse imaging embryo selection algorithms to predict implantation to demonstrate the need for the development of specific, in-house morphokinetic selection algorithms. Fertil Steril 2017;107:613–21.

43. Kostkova P, Brewer H, de Lusignan S, et al. Who Owns the Data? Open Data for Healthcare. Front Public Health 2016;4. Available at: http://journal.frontiersin.org/Article/10.3389/fpubh.2016.00007/abstract.

44. Murdoch B. Privacy and artificial intelligence: challenges for protecting health information in a new era. BMC Med Ethics 2021;22:122.

45. Davenport T, Kalakota R. The potential for artificial intelligence in healthcare. Future Healthc J 2019;6(2):94–8. PMID: 31363513; PMCID: PMC6616181.

46. Chow DJX, Wijesinghe P, Dholakia K, et al. Does artificial intelligence have a role in the IVF clinic? Reprod Fertil 2021;2(3):C29–34. PMID: 35118395; PMCID: PMC8801019.

Male Factor Infertility
What Every OB/GYN Should Know

Nihar Rama, BS[a], Hernan Lescay, MD[b],
Omer Raheem, MD, MSc, MCh, MRCS[b],*

KEYWORDS

- Male infertility • Azoospermia • Assisted reproductive technology
- Surgical sperm retrieval • Diagnostic evaluation

KEY POINTS

- Fertility is a couple's problem; therefore, initial infertility evaluation should include a parallel assessment of both female and male factor infertility.
- A thorough history, physical examination, and semen analysis are the cornerstone of evaluating male factor infertility and differentiating between the various possible etiologies.
- Common etiologies of male factor infertility, including causes of obstructive/nonobstructive azoospermia, asthenospermia, and more, are commonly associated with other health conditions with profound implications on both reproductive and overall men's health.
- The risk factors and causes of male infertility are not fully understood. Therefore, patients should be counseled about incorporating newer diagnostics and therapeutics options and their future implications on the management of male factor infertility.
- Various safe and effective surgical sperm retrieval techniques are available to enable assisted reproductive treatment including in vitro fertilization and/or intracytoplasmic sperm injection.

INTRODUCTION

Infertility is a complex condition that has challenging medical, psychological, economic, and social implications for both patients and clinicians. Based on the International Classification of Diseases (ICD-11), the World Health Organization (WHO) defines infertility as the failure to achieve a pregnancy after 12 months or more of regular unprotected sexual intercourse.[1] For women $\geq$ 35 years, failure to achieve pregnancy after 6 months or more of regular unprotected sexual intercourse warrants infertility evaluation.[2] Approximately 15% of couples with unknown fertility status

[a] Pritzker School of Medicine, University of Chicago, Chicago, IL, USA; [b] Department of Surgery, Section of Urology, University of Chicago Medicine, Chicago, IL, USA
* Corresponding author. Department of Surgery, Section of Urology, University of Chicago Medicine, 5841 S Maryland Avenue, MC6038, Chicago, IL 60637.
E-mail address: oraheem@bsd.uchicago.edu

Obstet Gynecol Clin N Am 50 (2023) 763–777
https://doi.org/10.1016/j.ogc.2023.08.001
0889-8545/23/© 2023 Elsevier Inc. All rights reserved.

are infertile after 1 year of unprotected intercourse, with male factor infertility solely responsible in ~30% of such couples and combined male and female factors present in an additional 20%.[3,4] A Global Burden of Disease survey reported in 2019 that infertility is on the rise, with the age-standardized prevalence of infertility in men increasing by 0.3% per year between 1990 and 2017.[5] Therefore, it is necessary for obstetrics and gynecology (OB/GYN) practitioners to be familiar with the standard evaluation and treatment available for male factor infertility given its implication in couple infertility.

Male factor infertility has a variety of identifiable and reversible causes, including but not limited to varicoceles, vas deferens obstruction, ejaculatory duct obstruction, and hypogonadotropic hypogonadism. Other causes of male infertility can be identified by abnormal semen analysis (SA). When abnormal SA is present without a clear etiology, male factor infertility is termed idiopathic. When female partner evaluation and SA do not explain infertility, the condition is termed unexplained.

Based on the WHOs ICD-11 definition of infertility, failure to achieve pregnancy after 12 months or more of unprotected intercourse (or 6 months if the female partner is more than age 35 years) should trigger comprehensive infertility evaluation and testing. However, several factors might suggest an earlier evaluation of a couple's fertility status is prudent. These factors include (1) risk factors for male infertility such as if a history of bilateral cryptorchidism and advanced paternal age (>40 years) are present[6]; (2) risk factors for female infertility such as advanced female age (>35 years) are present; and/ or (3) the couple questions the male partner's fertility potential. Providers should recognize that men with a history of previous fertility (ie, a male patient who has successfully conceived before) can acquire a new, secondary, male infertility factor. Therefore, a history of previous fertility should not preclude a male with concerns or risk factors for infertility from evaluation, and men with possible secondary infertility should be evaluated in the same way as men who have never initiated a pregnancy and are being evaluated for primary male factor infertility.[7]

In this comprehensive review, the authors discuss strategies OB/GYN providers can use to evaluate male factor infertility with the goals of identifying and differentiating between reversible etiologic conditions, irreversible conditions amenable to ART using the male partner's sperm, irreversible conditions for which donor insemination or adoption is more advisable, and other pathologies or etiologies with implications for the patient and their family.

BACKGROUND
Epidemiology of Male Infertility

Overall, infertility affects up to 15% of couples, with up to half of those having a male factor component to the infertility.[8] Unfortunately, much of the care for men undergoing infertility workups is outside the usual reimbursement systems, thus making it difficult to accurately track outcomes and epidemiologic data.[9] The National Survey of Family Growth found that up to 27% of men within infertile couples had never been evaluated for male factor infertility.[10] Early detection and management of male infertility can improve reproductive outcomes and prevent long-term psychological distress for affected couples.

Relationship Between Male Infertility and Overall Men's Health

Recent studies have identified male infertility as a biomarker for overall men's health, particularly urologic and cardiovascular health. For example, up to 6% of men evaluated for infertility have significant undiagnosed serious medical conditions, including testicular and/or prostate malignancies, even with normal SA.[11,12] Furthermore, numerous studies have suggested that infertile men have more comorbidities compared with their fertile controls; for example, men with abnormal semen parameters and azoospermia are more likely to have cancer compared with fertile men.[13–18] In half of cases, the underlying etiology of male infertility is known to be due to hypospadias, cryptorchidism, testosterone deficiency, or underlying genetic causes such as Klinefelter syndrome and cystic fibrosis. These male infertility-related medical conditions often warrant multidisciplinary counseling and management.[7]

Recent evidence suggests that advanced paternal age (> 40 years) could play a role in male factor infertility.[19] For example, the American Urologic Association (AUA) and the American Society for Reproductive Medicine (ASRM) Guidelines recommend that men of advanced paternal age whose offspring are at-risk for de novo intra- and intergenic germline mutations, sperm aneuploidy, chromosomal abnormalities, birth defects, and genetic conditions should be counseled on the absolute and relative risks for their offspring.

Access to Infertility Care

Although access to infertility care varies significantly by region or country, some common barriers include lack of insurance coverage, cost, cultural stigma, and geographic distance. In many low- and middle-income countries, access to infertility care is particularly limited due to a lack of resources and trained health care providers. Even in high-income countries with more robust health care systems, disparities in access persist, with marginalized communities and those with lower incomes facing significant barriers to care.

Interestingly, access to care and the characteristics of the fertility clinic in which a possibly infertile male is being evaluated are important considerations in evaluating and managing infertility. Variability in practice setting and size affect access to urologic care. Only about 11% of assisted reproductive technology (ART) fertility clinics have an on-site urologist, and variations in patient-facing educational materials can affect referral patterns to experts in male fertility evaluation. Therefore, OB/GYN providers should be aware of the importance of collaborating and partnering with reproductive urologists and andrologists to assist in evaluating and treating male factor infertility.[20] Many men seen in urology clinics have been referred by a reproductive endocrinologist and have already been treated with ART before an investigation into male factor infertility has started.[21]

Infertility can have significant financial costs for couples who are trying to conceive. Although WHO and the ASRM designate infertility as a disease, private insurance companies infrequently offer coverage for male infertility treatments. The Urologic Diseases in America project, which set out to collect male reproductive data epidemiologic data, found total expenditures of $17 million USD in 2000 for primary male infertility (excluding the cost of ART cycles, which is substantially more).[9] To date, there remain a paucity of epidemiologic data on male factor infertility, and thus, these numbers are expected to be an underestimate.

EVALUATION OF MALE INFERTILITY
Medical History

According to the AUA/ASRM guidelines, an evaluation of male infertility usually begins with a detailed medical, surgical, reproductive, and family history. This should include (1) coital frequency and timing; (2) duration of infertility and a history of prior fertility; (3) childhood illnesses (such as bilateral cryptorchidism, mumps orchitis, and other reproductive developmental histories); (3) past medical history (such as erectile dysfunction, premature ejaculation, Peyronie's disease, diabetes mellitus,[22] genetic disorders, upper respiratory diseases and testosterone, radiotherapy or chemotherapy exposure) and surgical history (including a history of prior vasectomy, inguinal hernia surgery, penetrating or blunt testicular trauma); (5) sexual history including any history of sexually transmitted infections; and (6) potential gonadal toxin exposure, including heat or cannabis.[23,24] In select cases or when referral to a reproductive urologist is not feasible in a timely fashion, OB/GYN providers may begin guideline-based fertility evaluation as appropriate and indicated including SA and laboratory hormonal evaluation.

Physical Examination

A comprehensive and directed physical examination includes (1) examination of body habitus, hair distribution, breast development, and other secondary sex characteristics; (2) external genitalia, urethral meatus, penile plaques, lesions, or deformities; (3) testes size (by examination or orchidometer) orientation and consistency; (4) presence or absence of vas deference and epididymis bilaterally (congenital bilateral absence of the vas deferens [CBAVD]); (5) presence or absence of varicoceles; (6) a digital rectal examination to evaluate for midline prostatic cysts or dilated seminal vesicles, which may assist in the diagnosis of ejaculatory duct obstruction.

Endocrine Hormonal Laboratory Testing

Endocrine and hormonal profile testing primarily focuses on evaluating the hypothalamic-pituitary-testicular axis (**Fig. 1**)[25] for several clinical scenarios, including (1) men with oligospermia (<10 million sperm/mL); (2) men with suspected impairment of their sexual function (including reduced libido); and (3) other clinical findings in the

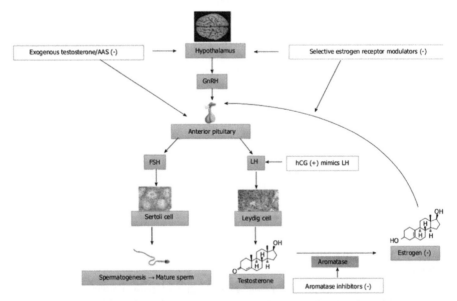

Fig. 1. Hypothalamic-pituitary-gonadal axis. (*From* Raheem et al., Sexual Medicine Reviews (with permission). Raheem OA, Chen T, Akula KP, et al. Efficacy of Non-Testosterone–Based Treatment in Hypogonadal Men: A Review. Sex Med Rev. 2021;9(3):381-392.)

history and examination that are suggestive of endocrine abnormalities. In addition, men with a history of erectile dysfunction, oligozoospermia, or azoospermia, hormonal testing should consist of an early morning measurement of serum follicle-stimulating hormone (FSH) which is normally less than approximately 7.6 IU/L and total testosterone (T) levels. A total T level of less than 300 ng/mL warrants further endocrine evaluation, including a second early morning measurement of total T and additional testing for free T, luteinizing hormone (LH), and prolactin. **Table 1**[26] summarizes the endocrine analysis for various conditions of hormonal imbalance in the hypothalamic-pituitary-testicular axis. For example, patients with hypogonadotropic hypogonadism will have a hormonal profile of low FSH, low LH, and low T. If endocrine analysis demonstrates low T with elevated FSH and LH, the patient might have primary testicular failure (hypergonadotropic hypogonadism) such as Klinefelter's syndrome. An endocrine analysis demonstrating low T with low FSH and LH levels is suggestive of secondary testicular failure (hypogonadotropic hypogonadism), as is the case in patients with Kallman's syndrome.

Table 2 outlines the endocrine hormonal profiles in men with azoospermia (no sperm counts that will be discussed in detail later in this review). For example, men with obstructive azoospermia will have normal FSH, LH, and T levels, whereas men with pre-testicular nonobstructive azoospermia have low FSH, LH, and T levels. It is important to consider endocrine physiology in evaluating men with suspected primary or secondary testicular failure. Therefore, to accurately diagnose the underlying etiology of male infertility, the history, clinical examination, and if indicated, the hormonal analysis should all be taken together into consideration.

Semen Analysis

SA is considered a critical test in the evaluation of male infertility according to the AUA/ASRM guidelines on male infertility. SA characteristics define the severity of the male factor infertility. Physicians should be aware that proper SA requires evaluation of *at least* two semen samples, ideally obtained at least 2 weeks apart, particularly if the first SA has abnormal parameters (WHO 2021 reference ranges in **Table 3**).[27] Before semen collection, patients should be provided with instructions to complete an

Table 1
Endocrine analysis for various conditions of hormonal imbalance in the hypothalamic-pituitary-testicular axis

Conditions	Follicle-Stimulating Hormone	Luteinizing Hormone	Testosterone	Prolactin
Normal spermatogenesis	Normal	Normal	Normal	Normal
Hypergonadotropic hypogonadism (primary testicular failure)	High	High	Low	Normal
Hypogonadotropic hypogonadism (secondary testicular failure)	Low	Low	Low	Normal
Abnormal spermatogenesis	High/normal	Normal	Normal/Low	Normal
Prolactin-secreting pituitary tumor	Normal/low	Normal/low	Low	High

Adapted from Raheem OA, Hsieh TC. Clinical Approaches to Male Factor Infertility. In: Palermo GD, Sills ES, eds. Intracytoplasmic Sperm Injection. Springer International Publishing; 2018:123 to 141. https://doi.org/10.1007/978-3-319-70497-5_9 (with permission).

Table 2
Endocrine analysis for men with azoospermia

Etiology	Follicle-Stimulating Hormone	Luteinizing Hormone	Testosterone
Obstructive azoospermia	Normal	Normal	Normal
Nonobstructive azoospermia; pre-testicular	Low	Low	Low
Nonobstructive azoospermia; exogenous testosterone	Low	Low	High
Nonobstructive azoospermia; testicular	High	High	Low

abstinence period of 2 to 5 days. One option for semen sample collection is seminal collection condoms designed without spermicidal agents that can be used to collect semen at home, keep the semen sample at room (or body) temperature during transport, and allow for examination within about 1 h of collection. Alternatively, patients can be instructed on masturbation (most common collection method) or coitus interruptus, though this latter method is not ideal as part of the ejaculate may be lost during collection.

In 2021, the WHO published the 6th edition of laboratory analysis of semen with updated reference values, as summarized in **Table 3**. It is imperative that clinicians recognize that if a male patient has an SA profile that falls within the normal reference ranges it is possible that they may still be infertile. Similarly, it is possible for fertile male patients to have semen variables outside of the reference range. Importantly, for providers providing assisted reproductive treatment (ART) including intrauterine insemination (IUI), an SA falling within the reference range may be adequate. However, the semen parameters necessary for unassisted conception are different from those required for ART. Clinicians should also be aware that the greater the number of abnormal SA parameters, the greater the likelihood of infertility.[28]

Computer-aided sperm analysis (CASA) is an effort to improve and standardize SA. CASA involves the use of microscopic or video imaging to determine specific semen parameters, including sperm motility and motion parameters such as velocity, speed, and head movement. These variables may be important factors in determining sperm fertility potential, but are not yet standard of care and have not replaced traditional SA for evaluating male infertility.[29] Artificial intelligence has also been used to streamline SA, with some evidence suggesting artificial intelligence can be a reliable diagnostic tool for evaluating male infertility.[30] Another advancement in SA is the development

Table 3
Semen analysis normal reference ranges by World Health Organization, 2021

Parameter	Normal Range
Volume (mL)	≥ 1.4
Sperm concentration (million/mL)	≥ 16
% Motility	≥ 42
% Progressive motility	≥ 30
% Strict morphology	≥ 4
Total sperm number (million)	≥ 39

From WHO laboratory manual for the examination of human semen, Sixth Edition. Published online 2021.

of home-based sperm testing systems based on microfluidics, smartphone technology, or antibody reactions with accuracy as high as 98%. Therefore, home-based sperm testing could be a practical and affordable way to screen for male infertility in at-risk populations.[31]

Providers should be aware that SA is an imperfect tool for evaluating male infertility. WHO manuals establishing reference values have been met with criticism surrounding the generalizability of the data given the limited representation of various racial/ethnic groups and the high degree of biological variation among individuals.[32] Therefore, providers should be scrutinous in their interpretation of SA and use multiple parameters to proceed through the diagnostic workup of possible male infertility.

Specific Semen Abnormalities

Azoospermia

Azoospermia is the absence of sperm from the semen. A diagnosis of azoospermia on SA is reached when a semen specimen is centrifuged at maximum speed for ~15 minutes with pellet examination.[33] It is also important for clinicians to be able to differentiate between azoospermia and anejaculation (failing to produce antegrade semen). Once a semen abnormality of azoospermia has been established, it is critically important for clinicians to determine the etiology to treat the cause of the azoospermia or, whenever possible, retrieve sperm to enable in vitro fertilization (IVF) and/or intracytoplasmic sperm injection (ICSI). Azoospermia accounts for about 10% to 15% of male factor infertility, and nearly 1% of all men are believed to be azoospermic.[34]

The etiologies of azoospermia are characterized as obstructive/post-testicular or nonobstructive/testicular. In obstructive azoospermia, there is adequate testicular sperm production in the setting of ductal obstruction. In nonobstructive azoospermia, sperm production is absent. The history, physical examination, hormonal studies, and imaging can help to differentiate between obstructive and nonobstructive azoospermia. It is worthwhile mentioning that semen volume, semen pH (alkaline vs acidic), and presence of fructose also aid in diagnosing azoospermia.

Oligospermia

Oligospermia is characterized by low sperm count. The WHO defines oligospermia as less than 15 million/mL.[23] Treatment options for oligospermia depend on the underlying cause and can include hormone therapy, surgery, lifestyle modifications, and assisted reproductive technologies such as IVF and ICSI.

Obstructive azoospermia

Obstructive azoospermia accounts for 40% of azoospermia. Causes of obstructive azoospermia include (1) structural causes, such as trauma from prior surgeries such as vasectomy, prior inguinal hernia repairs, prior hydrocele repairs, or orchiopexy; (2) nonstructural causes, such as CBAVD, sexually transmitted infections (namely chlamydia and gonorrhea); and (3) functional problems, including spinal injury, neurologic disease, and prior retroperitoneal disease. The endocrine profiles of men with obstructive azoospermia include normal FSH, LH, and testosterone (see **Table 2**), as well as normal testes on clinical examination and/or testicular ultrasound. If the cause of an obstructive azoospermia etiology for infertility is CBAVD, clinicians should be aware of the importance of cystic fibrosis testing. Up to 80% of men with CBAVD have mutations in the cystic fibrosis transmembrane regulator (*CFTR*) gene, and mutations in *CFTR* are prevalent in 20% of men with idiopathic epididymal obstruction and congenital unilateral absence of the vas deferens (CUAVD).[35–37] Therefore, the importance of genetic testing in the setting of evaluating and managing patients with these etiologies of obstructive azoospermia cannot be overstated. Furthermore, approximately 20% of men with CUAVD have ipsilateral renal agenesis due to abnormal mesonephric duct development with a slightly lower proportion in patients with CBAVD.[38–40] Therefore, renal ultrasound should be considered in patients with unilateral or bilateral absent vas deferens. Furthermore, for men diagnosed with CFTR mutation in the context of congenital absence of vas deference and obstructive azoospermia, it is recommended to evaluate their female partner for CFTR gene mutations before proceeding with future reproductive treatment.

Nonobstructive azoospermia

Nonobstructive azoospermia can be divided into classifications of pre-testicular and post-testicular nonobstructive azoospermia. Pre-testicular azoospermia, which presents with endocrine abnormalities suggestive of hypogonadotropic hypogonadism, has causes including Kallman's syndrome (patients presenting with anosmia and delayed puberty) and/or pituitary abnormalities (see **Table 2**). Testicular nonobstructive azoospermia, which will present with endocrine abnormalities suggestive of hypergonadotropic hypogonadism, involves impaired spermatogenesis (as is the case in the genetic disorder Klinefelter syndrome [47, XXY]), undescended testes and/or testicular torsion, varicoceles, testicular cancer, and gonadotoxins. Although pre- and post-testicular azoospermia is often treatable, testicular causes currently lack effective reversible management options.

Asthenospermia. Asthenospermia is a defect of sperm movement detected in SA by low sperm motility. The causes of asthenospermia are numerable and include genital tract infections associated with pyospermia, antisperm antibodies (ASAs), spermatozoal structural defects, ejaculatory duct obstruction, and varicoceles; asthenospermia can also be idiopathic. Additional laboratory testing for ASA can aid in the management of patients with asthenospermia. If ASAs are present, patients may be offered IUI or IVF/ICSI; alternatively, patients can be treated with immunosuppressive steroids, though the effectiveness of steroids is low and there is a risk of serious side effects.[41] If SA demonstrates low sperm motility in the setting of high viability, then disorders affecting sperm motility such as primary ciliary dyskinesia should be considered.[42]

Teratozoospermia

Teratozoospermia is a defect of sperm morphology. Sperm morphology assessment has evolved over the last several years with the recognition that even in semen from fertile men, sperm display a spectrum of what is considered normal morphology. However, sperm morphology is considered one of many indicators of sperm function and therefore has been used by some reproductive specialists to identify couples that might be better candidates for ICSI over IVF.[43] Globozoospermia is a structural defect, in which sperm have round heads, and this is often characterized by the absence of an acrosome and therefore impaired sperm function.[44] The fertility outcomes for male patients with globozoospermia are often poor.

Pyospermia

Pyospermia or leukocytospermia is the presence of white blood cells (WBCs) on SA and is defined by the presence of greater than 1×10^6 WBCs/mL under light microscope.[45] Pyospermia can result from infectious and noninfectious causes including toxins, varicocele, chronic prostatitis, and autoimmune disorders. The oxidative stress from an abnormal amount of inflammatory cells can affect the functionality of sperm, thus affecting fertilization capability.[45]

Genetic Testing

Given the association of azoospermia and severe oligospermia (<5 million) with genetic abnormalities, including mutations in the *CFTR* gene, Klinefelter syndrome (47, XXY), and the prevalence of microdeletions in the azoospermic factor (AZF) region of the long arm of the Y-chromosome (YCMD), genetic testing is strongly indicated for patients with azoospermia/severe oligospermia. Karyotyping and Y-chromosome microdeletion analysis can play a key role in the diagnostic workup and management of these patients. Specific to Y chromosome microdeletion (YCMD), there are three microdeletions (AZFa, AZFb, AZFc) on the long arm of the Y-chromosome that account for about 7% of cases of severe oligospermia/azoospermia in infertile male patients.[46] If an AZFc microdeletion is detected, microscopic testicular sperm extraction (TESE) (micro-TESE) might be indicated as micro-TESE yields a sperm retrieval rate of up to 70% in patients with AZFc microdeletions for future ART such as IVF and/or IVF/ICSI.[47] However, for patients with AZFa or AZFb microdeletions or combination, the chances of surgical sperm retrieval through micro-TESE are virtually nonexistent and donor sperm is highly recommended as per AUA/ASRM guidelines.

Given the close association of mutations in the *CFTR* gene and possible etiologies of obstructive azoospermia (CBAVD, CUAVD, and idiopathic epididymal obstruction), clinicians should consider referring patients with these conditions for genetic counseling. The AUA and ASRM recommend genetic testing to provide information on possible offspring transmission, which warrants the use of gene sequencing and carrier screening, including testing for the 5-thymidine (5T) allele of *CFTR*. If *CFTR* mutations are identified, preconception counseling should be offered to the patient and their partner to outline the risks of having a child with cystic fibrosis given the carrier status of the couple.

Karyotyping should be considered during genetic evaluation given the association of chromosomal abnormalities in patients with male infertility. In particular, Klinefelter syndrome (47, XXY) is the most common chromosomal abnormality seen in infertile men, accounting for approximately 15% of nonobstructive azoospermia. Klinefelter syndrome has an incidence of 1 in 600 phenotypic males and presents clinically with small, firm testicles, and diluted male secondary sex characteristics, including scant hair distribution.[48,49]

Specialized Testing

In select cases, conventional SA can be supplemented with additional sperm functional testing. For example, sperm function tests were developed after defective sperm-zona interaction was identified as the main reason for fertilization failure during IVF. The most commonly used assessment of sperm chromatin quality is through sperm DNA fragmentation testing, which can assess sperm chromatin structure and sperm chromatin dispersion.[50–52] Although the routine use of sperm DNA fragmentation testing is not recommended by the AUA/ASRM guideline and there is a lack of strict standardization and clear threshold values, in 2017, the Society for Translational Medicine published a clinical practice guideline for sperm DNA fragmentation testing outlining several clinical scenarios in which this testing may be warranted.[53] Sperm DNA fragmentation testing may be warranted in (1) patients with normal SA and a clinical grade 2 or 3 varicocele; (2) patients with borderline/abnormal SA and a clinical, grade 1 varicocele; (3) couples with unexplained infertility and/or recurrent pregnancy lost; (4) couples with IVF and/or ICSI failure; and (5) male patients with risk factors for male infertility, including environmental or occupational exposure to gonadotoxins[54] and lifestyle factors such as smoking,[55] alcohol consumption,[56] and recreational drug use.[57]

In certain cases of azoospermia, present vas deferens, and low semen volume SA, providers should consider ejaculatory dysfunction including retrograde ejaculation and usually recommend post-ejaculate urine analysis (PEU) to differentiate between retrograde ejaculation (with positive PEU) and other ejaculatory obstruction or dysfunction.[6]

Antisperm Antibodies

ASAs are antibodies that the body produces against sperm cells. They can be produced in response to a variety of factors including testicular trauma, vasectomy, vasectomy reversal, orchitis, cryptorchidism, neoplasm, and varicocele. ASAs affect fertility by decreasing sperm motility, agglutination, and penetration of the cervical mucus.[58]

Hyperviscosity Testing

Semen hyperviscosity refers to semen that has retained extra viscosity following the liquefication that physiologically occurs following ejaculation. Although the exact mechanisms contributing to semen hyperviscosity are incompletely understood, hyperviscous semen contributes to male infertility by negatively affecting sperm motility and semen quality.[59]

Testis Mapping and Biopsy

Traditionally, a testicular biopsy is considered to differentiate between obstructive and NOA, albeit the recent AUA/ASRM guidelines do not recommend a diagnostic testicular biopsy[60] owing to heterogeneity of spermatogenesis in men with azoospermia. On the contrary, fine-needle aspiration (FNA) testicular mapping has been popularized as an alternative diagnostic tool to stratify spermatogenesis in men with azoospermia based on the amount of sperm present or absent, early maturation arrest and Sertoli cell-only syndrome finding. FNA testis mapping consists of 12 to 18 (depending on testis size) fine-needle aspiration sites to extract the seminiferous tubules. These are then analyzed by a cytopathologist to assess the presence or absence of sperm and other findings as above. Mapping can aid in localizing sperm for future sperm retrieval techniques by identifying spermatogenesis loci for successful sperm retrieval and thus minimizing invasiveness and long-term sequelae, such as hypogonadism.

Imaging Tests

Scrotal ultrasound is typically not recommended in the initial evaluation of male infertility as per AUA/ASRM guidelines. This is because a thorough history and physical examination can typically identify the most common scrotal pathologies accounting for an infertility factor, including the presence of varicoceles, absent vasa deferens, and testicular masses. Scrotal ultrasound might be indicated in patients who are difficult to examine because of body habitus, undescended testis, testicular pain, or for patients with risk factors for malignancy and lately with the emergence of telehealth. Scrotal ultrasound can be helpful in examining spermatic cord vasculature. However scrotal ultrasound should not be routinely used to identify subclinical varicoceles as treatment of such varicoceles has little clinical utility. Traditionally, varicoceles are graded by size. Grade 0 varicoceles are subclinical and visible only via imaging; grade 1 varicoceles are palpable when patients perform the Valsalva maneuver; grade 2 varicoceles are palpable without the Valsalva maneuver; and grade 3 varicoceles are visible at rest.

Transrectal ultrasound (TRUS) is also not typically recommended as part of the initial workup for male infertility. However, in patients with possible ejaculatory duct obstruction per SA (with low semen volume, azoospermia, acidic SA, and fructose negative), dilated seminal vesicles (>2.5 cm), and/or midline prostatic cysts can be identified by TRUS.[61] In addition, cystoscopy evaluation of the lower urinary tract including midline utricle cysts, ejaculatory duct obstruction, strictures or stones, and urethral or prostate scarring or strictures can also be documented.

Pelvic and renal ultrasound and/or cross-sectional abdominal imaging with CT/MRI can be particularly helpful in patients with suspected pelvic cystic abnormalities or vasal agenesis given the high association of renal agenesis in disorders of vasal agenesis.[38]

Treatment

Although most of diagnosable causes of male infertility do not currently have effective treatments, about 20% of cases of male infertility are reversible and treatable conditions, including obstructive azoospermia, ejaculatory duct obstruction, prostatic midline cysts, gonadotropin deficiency, sexual function disorders, vasectomy reversal, varicoceles, and reversible effects from prior testosterone exposure, gonadotoxins, and sperm autoimmunity.[62]

Role of Supplements

Antioxidants are known to have protective effects against oxidative stress, which have been demonstrated in patients with sperm DNA damage and reduced motility, which lead to male infertility. The most studied antioxidants are vitamins E and C, coenzyme Q10, and selenium. A meta-analysis comparing seven small, randomized trials concluded a possible increase in live birth rates in those men taking antioxidants, but the investigators also concluded that this was based on low-quality evidence. Therefore, there remains a need for larger randomized control trials to evaluate the role of antioxidants in male infertility.[63]

Treatment options for patients with obstructive azoospermia include epididymal or testicular sperm retrieval for IVF/ICSI or surgical reconstruction. Both conventional and microdissection TESE are safe and effective options for patients eligible for sperm retrieval procedures.[64] Patients with nonobstructive azoospermia are less likely to benefit from sperm retrieval with success rates of about 50%. Therefore, men with nonobstructive azoospermia should be counseled on the options of donor sperm insemination or adoption.[65]

Varicoceles, or dilations of the pampiniform plexus venous vasculature within the spermatic cord, are present in healthy men about 15% of the time and in men with abnormal SA about 25% of the time.[6] Varicoceles can be repaired surgically or microsurgically, and surgical management is recommended for men with infertility with clinical varicoceles (grades 1–3), abnormal SA, and/or unexplained infertility with a female partner with no suspicion of female factor infertility. Varicocele repair can decrease sperm DNA fragmentation rates and reactive oxygen species. Livebirth outcomes following ART procedures are better for couples with male partners who received varicocele repair before ART.[66] Pregnancy and live birth rates have been shown to be 1.76-fold and 1.69-fold higher for men treated with varicocelectomy before ART, respectively.[66] Varicocele repair also seems to improve semen parameters, specifically sperm motility and total count.[67]

SUMMARY

Fertility evaluation should proceed in parallel for both male and female members of a couple to optimize fertility outcomes. Male factor infertility can be due to several causes and should be initially evaluated with a thorough history, physical examination, adequate SA, and when indicated, endocrine profile analysis. Abnormal SA findings include azoospermia (which warrants further workup to differentiate between obstructive and nonobstructive etiologies), asthenospermia, oligospermia, and teratozoospermia. Depending on the etiology of the male patient's etiology, assisted reproductive techniques may be offered to support the couple in their family planning goals. Given the complexity of managing patients with male infertility, OB/GYN providers should also leverage the expertise of reproductive urologists in evaluating and managing male factor infertility.

CLINICS CARE POINTS

- Initial infertility evaluation should include a parallel assessment of both female and male factor infertility.
- Evaluation of male infertility should include a thorough history, physical examination, and semen analysis, with high-quality semen analysis requiring at least two assessments spaced ideally at least 2 weeks apart.
- Men with infertility and/or abnormal semen parameters should be counseled on possible associated conditions and health risks associated with their reproductive condition.
- Patients should be counseled that the risk factors and causes for male infertility are incompletely understood and that new data are emerging to support future recommendations regarding the evaluation and management of male factor infertility.

DISCLOSURE

This research did not receive any grants or funding from funding agencies in the public, commercial, or not-for-profit sectors.

REFERENCES

1. International Classiciation of Diseases. 11th Revision (ICD-11). Baltimore, MD: Springer International publishing; 2019.
2. Definitions of infertility and recurrent pregnancy loss: a committee opinion. Fertil Steril 2020;113(3):533–5.
3. Louis JF, Thoma ME, Sørensen DN, et al. The prevalence of couple infertility in the United States from a male perspective: evidence from a nationally representative sample. Andrology 2013;1(5):741–8.
4. Kumar N, Singh A. Trends of male factor infertility, an important cause of infertility: A review of literature. J Hum Reprod Sci 2015;8(4):191.
5. Sun H, Gong TT, Jiang YT, et al. Global, regional, and national prevalence and disability-adjusted life-years for infertility in 195 countries and territories, 1990–2017: results from a global burden of disease study, 2017. Aging 2019;11(23): 10952–91.
6. Agarwal A, Baskaran S, Parekh N, et al. Male infertility. Lancet 2021;397(10271): 319–33.
7. Schlegel PN, Sigman M, Collura B, et al. Diagnosis and Treatment of Infertility in Men: AUA/ASRM Guideline Part I. J Urol 2021;205(1):36–43.
8. Bak CW, Song SH, Yoon TK, et al. Natural course of idiopathic oligozoospermia: Comparison of mild, moderate and severe forms: Different fates of oligozoospermia. Int J Urol 2010;17(11):937–43.

9. Meacham RB, Joyce GF, Wise M, et al. Urologic Diseases in America Project. Male Infertility. J Urol 2007;177(6):2058–66.
10. Eisenberg ML, Lathi RB, Baker VL, et al. Frequency of the male infertility evaluation: data from the national survey of family growth. J Urol 2013;189(3):1030–4.
11. Honig SC, Lipshultz LI, Jarow J. Significant medical pathology uncovered by a comprehensive male infertility evaluation. Fertil Steril 1994;62(5):1028–34.
12. Kolettis PN, Sabanegh ES. Significant medical pathology discovered during a male infertility evaluation. J Urol 2001;166(1):178–80.
13. Glazer C, Bonde J, Eisenberg M, et al. Male Infertility and Risk of Nonmalignant Chronic Diseases: A Systematic Review of the Epidemiological Evidence. Semin Reprod Med 2017;35(03):282–90.
14. Eisenberg ML, Betts P, Herder D, et al. Increased risk of cancer among azoospermic men. Fertil Steril 2013;100(3):681–5.e1.
15. Raman JD, Nobert CF, Goldstein M. Increased incidence of testicular cancer in men presenting with infertility and abnormal semen analysis. J Urol 2005; 174(5):1819–22.
16. Mancini M, Carmignani L, Gazzano G, et al. High prevalence of testicular cancer in azoospermic men without spermatogenesis. Hum Reprod 2007;22(4):1042–6.
17. Hanson HA, Anderson RE, Aston KI, et al. Subfertility increases risk of testicular cancer: evidence from population-based semen samples. Fertil Steril 2016; 105(2):322–8.e1.
18. Negri L, Benaglia R, Fiamengo B, et al. Cancer Risk in Male Factor-infertility. Placenta 2008;29:178–83.
19. Londero AP, Rossetti E, Pittini C, et al. Maternal age and the risk of adverse pregnancy outcomes: a retrospective cohort study. BMC Pregnancy Childbirth 2019; 19(1):261.
20. Shabto JM, Patil D, Poulose K, et al. Access to Care for Infertile Men: Referral Patterns of Fertility Clinics in the United States. Urology 2022;166:152–8.
21. Samplaski MK, Smith JF, Lo KC, et al. Reproductive endocrinologists are the gatekeepers for male infertility care in North America: results of a North American survey on the referral patterns and characteristics of men presenting to male infertility specialists for infertility investigations. Fertil Steril 2019;112(4):657–62.
22. Raheem OA, Hehemann MC, Rogers MJ, et al. Does Type 1 Diabetes Affect Male Infertility: Type 1 Diabetes Exchange Registry-Based Analysis. Société Int D'Urologie J. 2021;2(3):139–43.
23. Rajanahally S, Raheem O, Rogers M, et al. The relationship between cannabis and male infertility, sexual health, and neoplasm: a systematic review. Andrology 2019;7(2):139–47.
24. Hehemann MC, Raheem OA, Rajanahally S, et al. Evaluation of the impact of marijuana use on semen quality: a prospective analysis. Ther Adv Urol 2021; 13. 175628722110324.
25. Raheem OA, Chen T, Akula KP, et al. Efficacy of Non-Testosterone–Based Treatment in Hypogonadal Men: A Review. Sex Med Rev 2021;9(3):381–92.
26. Raheem OA, Hsieh TC. Clinical Approaches to Male Factor Infertility. In: Palermo GD, Sills ES, editors. Intracytoplasmic sperm injection. Cham: Springer International Publishing; 2018. p. 123–41. https://doi.org/10.1007/978-3-319-70497-5_9.
27. WHO laboratory manual for the examination of human semen, Sixth Edition. Published online 2021.
28. Guzick DS, Overstreet JW, Factor-Litvak P, et al. Sperm Morphology, Motility, and Concentration in Fertile and Infertile Men. N Engl J Med 2001;345(19):1388–93.

29. Larsen L. Computer-assisted semen analysis parameters as predictors for fertility of men from the general population. Hum Reprod 2000;15(7):1562–7.
30. Agarwal A, Henkel R, Huang C, et al. Automation of human semen analysis using a novel artificial intelligence optical microscopic technology. Andrologia 2019; 51(11). https://doi.org/10.1111/and.13440.
31. Yu S, Rubin M, Geevarughese S, et al. Emerging technologies for home-based semen analysis. Andrology 2018;6(1):10–9.
32. Esteves SC. Clinical relevance of routine semen analysis and controversies surrounding the 2010 World Health Organization criteria for semen examination. Int Braz J Urol 2014;40(4):433–53.
33. Corea M, Campagnone J, Sigman M. The diagnosis of azoospermia depends on the force of centrifugation. Fertil Steril 2005;83(4):920–2.
34. Cocuzza M, Alvarenga C, Pagani R. The epidemiology and etiology of azoospermia. Clinics 2013;68:15–26.
35. Mak V. Proportion of Cystic Fibrosis Gene Mutations Not Detected by Routine Testing in Men With Obstructive Azoospermia. JAMA 1999;281(23):2217.
36. Chillón M, Casals T, Mercier B, et al. Mutations in the Cystic Fibrosis Gene in Patients with Congenital Absence of the Vas Deferens. N Engl J Med 1995;332(22): 1475–80.
37. Yu J, Chen Z, Ni Y, et al. CFTR mutations in men with congenital bilateral absence of the vas deferens (CBAVD): a systemic review and meta-analysis. Hum Reprod 2012;27(1):25–35.
38. Schlegel PN, Shin D, Goldstein M. Urogenital Anomalies in Men with Congenital Absence of the Vas Deferens. J Urol 1996;155(5):1644–8.
39. Weiske WH, Sälzler N, Schroeder-Printzen I, et al. Clinical findings in congenital absence of the vasa deferentia. Andrologia 2000;32(1):13–8.
40. Kolettis PN, Sandlow JI. Clinical and genetic features of patients with congenital unilateral absence of the vas deferens. Urology 2002;60(6):1073–6.
41. Gupta S, Sharma R, Agarwal A, et al. Antisperm Antibody Testing: A Comprehensive Review of Its Role in the Management of Immunological Male Infertility and Results of a Global Survey of Clinical Practices. World J Mens Health 2022; 40(3):380.
42. Vanaken GJ, Bassinet L, Boon M, et al. Infertility in an adult cohort with primary ciliary dyskinesia: phenotype–gene association. Eur Respir J 2017;50(5): 1700314.
43. Pisarska MD, Casson PR, Cisneros PL, et al. Fertilization after standard in vitro fertilization versus intracytoplasmic sperm injection in subfertile males using sibling oocytes. Fertil Steril 1999;71(4):627–32.
44. Dam AHDM, Feenstra I, Westphal JR, et al. Globozoospermia revisited. Hum Reprod Update 2007;13(1):63–75.
45. Velez D, Ohlander S, Niederberger C. Pyospermia: background and controversies. FS Rep 2021;2(1):2–6.
46. Stahl PJ, Masson P, Mielnik A, et al. A decade of experience emphasizes that testing for Y microdeletions is essential in American men with azoospermia and severe oligozoospermia. Fertil Steril 2010;94(5):1753–6.
47. Krausz C, Riera-Escamilla A. Genetics of male infertility. Nat Rev Urol 2018;15(6): 369–84.
48. Yoshida A, Miura K, Shirai M. Cytogenetic Survey of 1,007 Infertile Males. Urol Int 1997;58(3):166–76.
49. Ghorbel M, Gargouri Baklouti S, Ben Abdallah F, et al. Chromosomal defects in infertile men with poor semen quality. J Assist Reprod Genet 2012;29(5):451–6.

50. Ward WS. Function of sperm chromatin structural elements in fertilization and development. Mol Hum Reprod 2010;16(1):30–6.
51. Oleszczuk K, Giwercman A, Bungum M. Intra-individual variation of the sperm chromatin structure assay DNA fragmentation index in men from infertile couples. Hum Reprod 2011;26(12):3244–8.
52. Agarwal A, Panner Selvam MK, Baskaran S, et al. Sperm DNA damage and its impact on male reproductive health: a critical review for clinicians, reproductive professionals and researchers. Expert Rev Mol Diagn 2019;19(6):443–57.
53. Agarwal A, Cho CL, Majzoub A, et al. The Society for Translational Medicine: clinical practice guidelines for sperm DNA fragmentation testing in male infertility. Transl Androl Urol 2017;6(S4):S720–33.
54. Ma Y, He X, Qi K, et al. Effects of environmental contaminants on fertility and reproductive health. J Environ Sci 2019;77:210–7.
55. Sharma R, Harlev A, Agarwal A, et al. Cigarette Smoking and Semen Quality: A New Meta-analysis Examining the Effect of the 2010 World Health Organization Laboratory Methods for the Examination of Human Semen. Eur Urol 2016;70(4):635–45.
56. Ricci E, Al Beitawi S, Cipriani S, et al. Semen quality and alcohol intake: a systematic review and meta-analysis. Reprod Biomed Online 2017;34(1):38–47.
57. Fronczak CM, Kim ED, Barqawi AB. The Insults of Illicit Drug Use on Male Fertility. J Androl 2012;33(4):515–28.
58. Bozhedomov VA, Lipatova NA, Alexeev RA, et al. The role of the antisperm antibodies in male infertility assessment after microsurgical varicocelectomy. Andrology 2014;2(6):847–55.
59. Agarwal A. Semen hyperviscosity causes consequences and cures. Front Biosci 2013;E5(1):224–31.
60. Kapadia AA, Walsh TJ. Testicular Mapping: A Roadmap to Sperm Retrieval in Nonobstructive Azoospermia? Male Infertil 2020;47(2):157–64.
61. Engin G, Celtik M, Sanli O, et al. Comparison of transrectal ultrasonography and transrectal ultrasonography-guided seminal vesicle aspiration in the diagnosis of the ejaculatory duct obstruction. Fertil Steril 2009;92(3):964–70.
62. Barak S, Baker HWG. Clinical Management of Male Infertility. In: Feingold KR, Anawalt B, Blackman MR, et al., eds Endotext. MDText.com, Inc.; 2000 Accessed January 27, 2023. Available at: http://www.ncbi.nlm.nih.gov/books/NBK279160/.
63. Smits RM, Mackenzie-Proctor R, Yazdani A, et al. Antioxidants for male subfertility. Cochrane Database Syst Rev 2019;3(3):CD007411.
64. Corona G, Minhas S, Giwercman A, et al. Sperm recovery and ICSI outcomes in men with non-obstructive azoospermia: a systematic review and meta-analysis. Hum Reprod Update 2019;25(6):733–57.
65. Management of nonobstructive azoospermia: a committee opinion. Fertil Steril 2018;110(7):1239–45.
66. Kirby EW, Wiener LE, Rajanahally S, et al. Undergoing varicocele repair before assisted reproduction improves pregnancy rate and live birth rate in azoospermic and oligospermic men with a varicocele: a systematic review and meta-analysis. Fertil Steril 2016;106(6):1338–43.
67. Baazeem A, Belzile E, Ciampi A, et al. Varicocele and Male Factor Infertility Treatment: A New Meta-analysis and Review of the Role of Varicocele Repair. Eur Urol 2011;60(4):796–808.

UNITED STATES POSTAL SERVICE ®

Statement of Ownership, Management, and Circulation (All Periodicals Publications Except Requester Publications)

1. Publication Title
OBSTETRICS AND GYNECOLOGY CLINICS OF NORTH AMERICA

2. Publication Number
000 – 276

3. Filing Date
9/18/2023

4. Issue Frequency
MAR, JUN, SEP, DEC

5. Number of Issues Published Annually
4

6. Annual Subscription Price
$355.00

7. Complete Mailing Address of Known Office of Publication (Not printer) (Street, city, county, state, and ZIP+4®)
ELSEVIER INC.
230 Park Avenue, Suite 800
New York, NY 10169

Contact Person
Malathi Samayan

Telephone (Include area code)
91-44-4299-4507

8. Complete Mailing Address of Headquarters or General Business Office of Publisher (Not printer)
ELSEVIER INC.
230 Park Avenue, Suite 800
New York, NY 10169

9. Full Names and Complete Mailing Addresses of Publisher, Editor, and Managing Editor (Do not leave blank)

Publisher (Name and complete mailing address)
DOLORES MELONI, ELSEVIER INC.
1600 JOHN F KENNEDY BLVD. SUITE 1600
PHILADELPHIA, PA 19103-2899

Editor (Name and complete mailing address)
KERRY HOLLAND, ELSEVIER INC.
1600 JOHN F KENNEDY BLVD. SUITE 1600
PHILADELPHIA, PA 19103-2899

Managing Editor (Name and complete mailing address)
PATRICK MANLEY, ELSEVIER INC.
1600 JOHN F KENNEDY BLVD. SUITE 1600
PHILADELPHIA, PA 19103-2899

10. Owner (Do not leave blank. If the publication is owned by a corporation, give the name and address of the corporation immediately followed by the names and addresses of all stockholders owning or holding 1 percent or more of the total amount of stock. If not owned by a corporation, give the names and addresses of the individual owners. If owned by a partnership or other unincorporated firm, give its name and address as well as those of each individual owner. If the publication is published by a nonprofit organization, give its name and address.)

Full Name	Complete Mailing Address
WHOLLY OWNED SUBSIDIARY OF REED/ELSEVIER, US HOLDINGS	1600 JOHN F KENNEDY BLVD. SUITE 1600 PHILADELPHIA, PA 19103-2899

11. Known Bondholders, Mortgagees, and Other Security Holders Owning or Holding 1 Percent or More of Total Amount of Bonds, Mortgages, or Other Securities. If none, check box ▶ ☐ None

Full Name	Complete Mailing Address
N/A	

12. Tax Status (For completion by nonprofit organizations authorized to mail at nonprofit rates) (Check one)
The purpose, function, and nonprofit status of this organization and the exempt status for federal income tax purposes:
☒ Has Not Changed During Preceding 12 Months
☐ Has Changed During Preceding 12 Months (Publisher must submit explanation of change with this statement)

PS Form **3526**, July 2014 [Page 1 of 4 (see instructions page 4)] PSN: 7530-01-000-9931 PRIVACY NOTICE: See our privacy policy on www.usps.com.

13. Publication Title
OBSTETRICS AND GYNECOLOGY CLINICS OF NORTH AMERICA

14. Issue Date for Circulation Data Below
JUNE 2023

15. Extent and Nature of Circulation

		Average No. Copies Each Issue During Preceding 12 Months	No. Copies of Single Issue Published Nearest to Filing Date
a. Total Number of Copies (Net press run)		160	146
b. Paid Circulation (By Mail and Outside the Mail)	(1) Mailed Outside-County Paid Subscriptions Stated on PS Form 3541 (Include paid distribution above nominal rate, advertiser's proof copies, and exchange copies)	64	72
	(2) Mailed In-County Paid Subscriptions Stated on PS Form 3541 (Include paid distribution above nominal rate, advertiser's proof copies, and exchange copies)	0	0
	(3) Paid Distribution Outside the Mails Including Sales Through Dealers and Carriers, Street Vendors, Counter Sales, and Other Paid Distribution Outside USPS®	82	59
	(4) Paid Distribution by Other Classes of Mail Through the USPS (e.g., First-Class Mail®)	11	12
c. Total Paid Distribution (Sum of 15b (1), (2), (3), and (4))	▶	157	143
d. Free or Nominal Rate Distribution (By Mail and Outside the Mail)	(1) Free or Nominal Rate Outside-County Copies included on PS Form 3541	2	2
	(2) Free or Nominal Rate In-County Copies Included on PS Form 3541	0	0
	(3) Free or Nominal Rate Copies Mailed at Other Classes Through the USPS (e.g., First-Class Mail)	0	0
	(4) Free or Nominal Rate Distribution Outside the Mail (Carriers or other means)	1	1
e. Total Free or Nominal Rate Distribution (Sum of 15d (1), (2), (3) and (4))	▶	3	3
f. Total Distribution (Sum of 15c and 15e)	▶	160	146
g. Copies not Distributed (See Instructions to Publishers #4 (page 83))	▶	0	0
h. Total (Sum of 15f and g)	▶	160	146
i. Percent Paid (15c divided by 15f times 100)	▶	97.97%	97.95%

* If you are claiming electronic copies, go to line 16 on page 3. If you are not claiming electronic copies, skip to line 17 on page 3.

PS Form **3526**, July 2014 (Page 2 of 4)

16. Electronic Copy Circulation

	Average No. Copies Each Issue During Preceding 12 Months	No. Copies of Single Issue Published Nearest to Filing Date
a. Paid Electronic Copies ▶		
b. Total Paid Print Copies (Line 15c) + Paid Electronic Copies (Line 16a) ▶		
c. Total Print Distribution (Line 15f) + Paid Electronic Copies (Line 16a) ▶		
d. Percent Paid (Both Print & Electronic Copies) (16b divided by 16c × 100) ▶		

☒ I certify that 50% of all my distributed copies (electronic and print) are paid above a nominal price.

17. Publication of Statement of Ownership

☒ If the publication is a general publication, publication of this statement is required. Will be printed in the DECEMBER 2023 issue of this publication. ☐ Publication not required.

18. Signature and Title of Editor, Publisher, Business Manager, or Owner

Malathi Samayan

Malathi Samayan - Distribution Controller

Date 9/18/2023

I certify that all information furnished on this form is true and complete. I understand that anyone who furnishes false or misleading information on this form or who omits material or information requested on the form may be subject to criminal sanctions (including fines and imprisonment) and/or civil sanctions (including civil penalties).

PS Form **3526**, July 2014 (Page 3 of 4) PRIVACY NOTICE: See our privacy policy on www.usps.com

Moving?

Make sure your subscription moves with you!

To notify us of your new address, find your **Clinics Account Number** (located on your mailing label above your name), and contact customer service at:

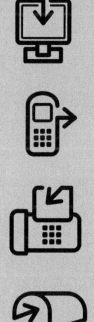

Email: journalscustomerservice-usa@elsevier.com

800-654-2452 (subscribers in the U.S. & Canada)
314-447-8871 (subscribers outside of the U.S. & Canada)

Fax number: 314-447-8029

Elsevier Health Sciences Division
Subscription Customer Service
3251 Riverport Lane
Maryland Heights, MO 63043

Printed and bound by CPI Group (UK) Ltd, Croydon, CR0 4YY

08/05/2025

01864749-0008